Speech Therapy Aphasia Rehabilitation
STAR
Workbook

Receptive Language

Amanda P. Anderson M.S. CCC-SLP

Cover Photograph: Courtesy of the European Southern Observatory

i

About The Author:

Amanda Anderson is a Speech-Language Pathologist and has worked in a combination of assisted living, skilled nursing, outpatient, and acute care settings with adults. She specializes in stroke rehabilitation in both speech, language and swallowing disorders. She graduated with honors from Davidson College in Davidson, North Carolina. She received her Master's Degree in Speech-Language Pathology from the University of Hawaii. She holds her certificate of clinical competence from the American Speech-Language-Hearing Association in Speech-Language Pathology.

She is the author of *Speech Therapy Aphasia Rehabilitation *STAR* Workbook for Expressive and Written Language.* She has also edited a war memoir for her late grandfather, Louis Lauria, *Running Wire on the Front Lines* which was published by McFarland. She created this aphasia workbook for receptive language for both Speech-Language Pathologists and stroke survivors and their caregivers to use to improve communication.

Table of Contents

Take Action!

I wrote these aphasia workbooks for several of my patients' whose Medicare part B benefits no longer covered speech therapy. All too often, individuals who have a stroke resulting in aphasia also need physical therapy. Currently, there is a therapy cap of $1,900 for both speech-language pathology and physical therapy combined. Rarely is this enough to support patients through a full physical and speech-language recovery.

Please take action! Contact your representatives and let them know how the therapy caps have negatively impacted you. The American Speech-Language and Hearing Association has an easy form to email to your members of Congress. Visit their website asha.org and under the advocacy tab you will find the take action section to contact congress to repeal the Medicare Part B caps. Currently, the link to the form is:

http://takeaction.asha.org/asha2/issues/alert/?alertid=62421566

Forward

by: Dr. Jodi Dodds, Vascular Neurologist

Language and communication enable us to function as a society. We exchange information with our families, our neighbors, our colleagues, those with whom we are involved in transactions. We find the right things to say, and when there is nothing that can be said, we listen empathetically in understanding of what others convey to us in conversation. We laugh at the humor in jokes, and we feel angry when hurtful words come our way. Spoken and comprehended language enhances what we feel hundreds of times each day.

When I first began treating stroke patients as a vascular neurologist, I thought the greatest challenges I would face would involve physical disabilities: weakness in an arm or a leg, or difficulties people would face with balance when ambulating. What I quickly learned was that aphasia, or disruptions in expressed or interpreted language, can be just as disabling as a severe physical limitation. Patients with aphasia have shared similar stories with me. These are stories of efforts to formulate comments during a family dinner discussion, only to find that once the language is processed and ready to be spoken, the conversation has moved on to a different topic. Patients claim they experience complex thoughts and ideas, but find frustration when their words fail them. I have heard tales from English teachers who have read one book each week for 30 years, only to find that after their strokes it may take months to complete a book, and retaining what they have read may require reading and rereading the same paragraphs three or four times.

One of the valuable evidence-based resources for patients struggling with aphasia is speech therapy as part of their rehabilitation plan. If they quality with their particular medical insurance plan, in particular if an accompanying physical deficit is also present after a brain injury, a patient with aphasia may start his or her rehabilitation journey at an acute rehabilitation facility with daily therapy in an attempt to optimize early recovery. After discharging from acute rehabilitation, patients will then usually undergo speech therapy either at home or in an outpatient clinic, although less frequently (perhaps 2-3 times each week). Once a patient is deemed to have "plateaued," meaning the patient is no longer demonstrating objective, measurable progress, he or she is often discharged from speech therapy as this may no longer be covered under the patient's medical insurance. Another common scenario is that a patient may receive a specified number of speech therapy visits under a particular health plan, and once these are exhausted, formal speech therapy stops.

My advice to patients in these scenarios who felt they could still make further progress and were motivated to continue working independently to rehabilitate themselves used to be fairly limited. I would advise them to read as much as possible, and to attempt to discuss what they were reading with friends or family members. Read the newspaper, I would recommend, circle words that are unfamiliar, and ask a designated family member each day what they are, or try to utilize a dictionary. Engage in conversation with someone who is calm and patient, and continue to practice regular dialogue. Babies do not learn to speak and comprehend language overnight, but over years, and recovering from aphasia following a significant brain injury usually does not happen overnight either.

I first met Amanda Anderson, SLP, in 2011. She often worked with stroke patients in her career as a speech language pathologist, and had the same feelings of concern for patients who were discharged from speech therapy but were still motivated to progress further with language recovery. In 2013, she brought a copy of her first aphasia workbook, *Speech Therapy Aphasia Rehabilitation Workbook: Expressive and Written Language*, to the neurology clinic where I see patients, and I was quickly impressed. I showed the book to several patients, who purchased it and started working through the exercises. They returned for follow up visits and wanted to know if there was a second volume available. Their families commented that the book motivated them to continue with engagement in their own recoveries. I am thrilled to finally have a useful, affordable option to offer patients with aphasia who want to do more.

Ms. Anderson has now completed a second volume, *Speech Therapy Aphasia Rehabilitation *STAR* Workbook II: Receptive Language*, focusing largely on receptive (or understood) language deficits, and opening independent language rehabilitation to a new group of patients afflicted with aphasia.

I am personally grateful for the opportunity to offer my patients an additional tool in their aphasia recovery journey, and recommend both of these workbooks to any physician or medical provider treating stroke patients or populations of patients who have sustained brain injury with residual aphasia.

Jodi A. Dodds, MD
Vascular Neurologist
Charlotte, North Carolina

Introduction

Receptive aphasia is a result of damage to the part of the brain that controls language comprehension. Typically, the posterior portion of the temporal lobe on the left hemisphere controls language comprehension and is called Wernicke's area. Damage to this part of the brain can be caused by a stroke, brain tumor, infection, brain injury, aneurism or dementia.

People with receptive aphasia have difficulty understanding everyday conversation and require additional time to process spoken and written language. Background noise, distractions and multiple speakers make comprehension increasingly difficult. Individuals with receptive aphasia can have difficulty with understanding speech, especially at a fast rate. Receptive aphasia also impairs an individual's ability to understand inferences and someone with aphasia may often only understand literal meanings.

This workbook combines exercises for individuals with severe receptive aphasia and challenging activities for people with mild deficits. Many of the exercises require limited expressive language to indicate comprehension. Often people with receptive aphasia also have expressive language deficits. The exercises give the patient the opportunity to point to or circle the correct answer instead of solely relying on spoken replies. Sometimes people with receptive aphasia may say "yes" even though they mean and are thinking "no". Repetition of both the question and the response may be necessary to ensure comprehension of each exercise.

To start, make sure to read the questions slowly and clearly. Limit all distractions and try to work in a quiet room with limited visual stimuli. Once the exercises become easier, you can add distractions. Work with the door open, keep the TV on, and read at a faster pace to continue to challenge the patient's receptive abilities.

Matching: This section is meant for individuals with severe receptive aphasia. The exercises start at the single word level and have the patient match the picture to the correct word. The choices increase as the section continues as does the difficulty level. The simple stark black and white images help improve the patient's ability to focus on comprehending each image.

Yes/No questions: The workbook contains multiple types of yes/no questions to target a variety of comprehension abilities. This section covers personal knowledge, comprehension of both concrete and abstract concepts as well as inferences. If someone has expressive deficits, have them point to or circle yes or no and then say the answer aloud once they have confirmed it visually.

The "Wh" questions all provided choices and are not open ended questions to accommodate patients with expressive language deficits. If your patient has strong expressive language skills, you can omit the choices to increase the difficulty level.

One Step and Multiple Step Directions: This group of questions is designed to give the patient the opportunity to demonstrate and improve comprehension through movement and gestures. The questions take into consideration that the patient may have hemiparesis as a result of a stroke. Rarely do the directions require an individual to use both arms or legs. Some of the multiple step directions may need modification depending on the setting where you are working. Some questions are geared towards a hospital or skilled nursing room while others use materials found in assisted living or an individual's home. The multiple step directions with materials and images increase in difficulty level and are appropriate for mild to moderate receptive aphasia.

The next sections of the workbook concentrate on the patients ability to comprehend details starting at the sentence level progressing up to short stories. These questions can be both read aloud and given to the patient to read. Start with whichever is easier for the patient. Repeat the sentences as often as needed as well as the question. As progress is made, reduce the repetition and increase the speed and distractions.

The final section of the workbook focuses on cognitive processing skills. The calculation questions are meant to be challenging. Repeat the question and even help your patient write down the problems to work them out on paper if needed. These questions utilize the brain's ability to comprehend multiple steps required to complete word problems as well as attention, cognitive processing, and working memory skills.

Speech therapy helps the brain form new neurological connections after an area of the brain has sustained damage. By building on existing skills, therapy can increase ability levels to increase receptive language function. Gestures, repetition, pacing and limiting distractions are strategies that can help improve receptive language function. Motivation, repetition and strong caregiver support are all factors that will contribute to steady recovery of receptive language skills.

Matching: Circle the word that matches the picture.

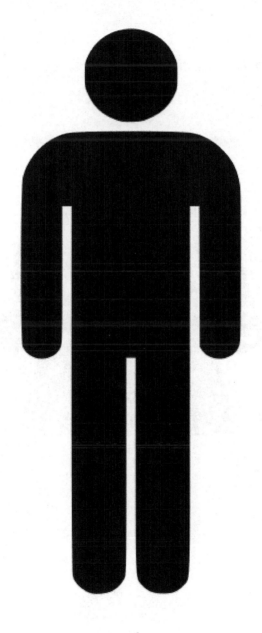

Man   Woman

Matching: Circle the word that matches the picture.

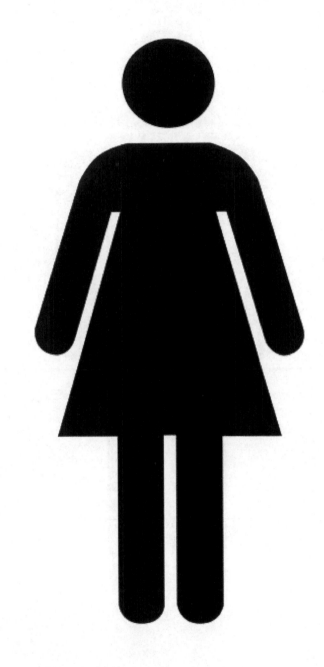

Man   Woman

Matching: Circle the word that matches the picture.

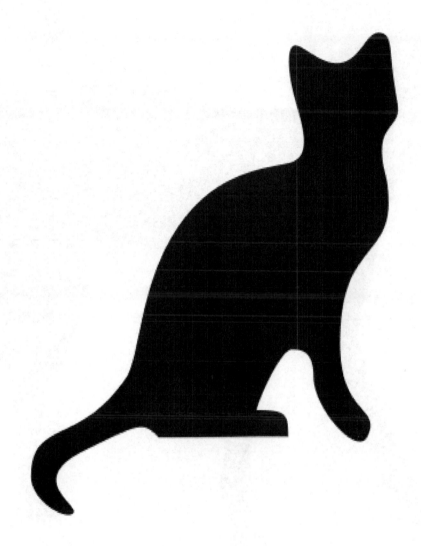

Cat   Dog

Matching: Circle the word that matches the picture.

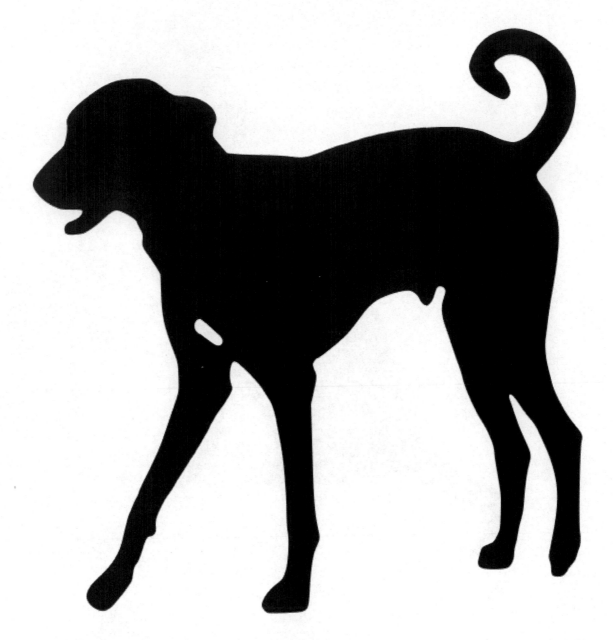

iii

Cat   Dog

Matching: Circle the word that matches the picture.

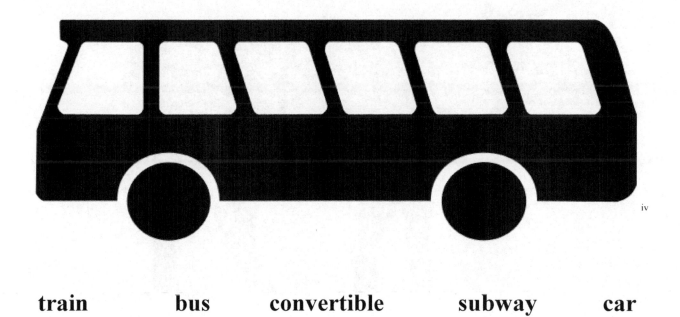

train bus convertible subway car

lizard snake tadpole frog fish

Matching: Circle the word that matches the picture.

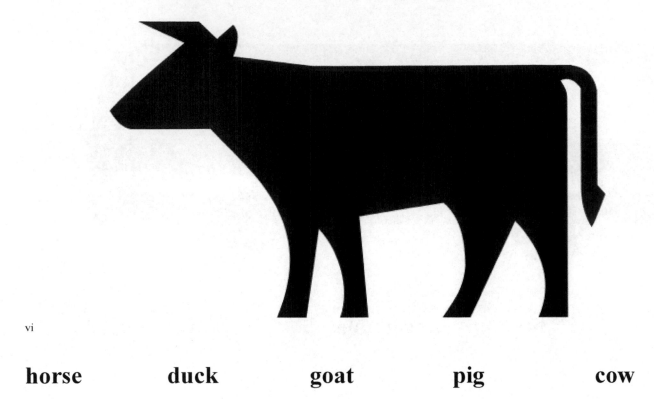

vi

horse   **duck**   **goat**   **pig**   **cow**

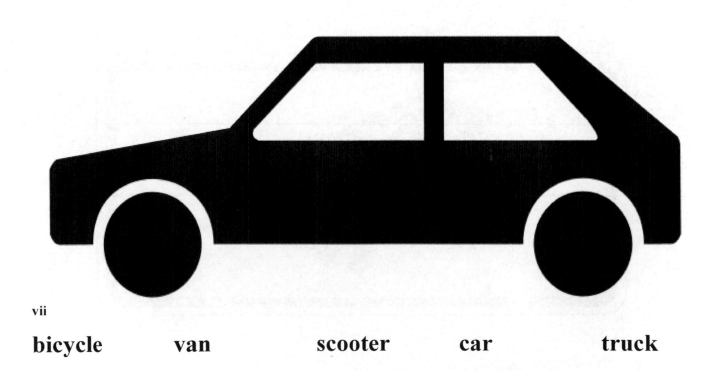

vii

bicycle   **van**   **scooter**   **car**   **truck**

Matching: Circle the word that matches the picture.

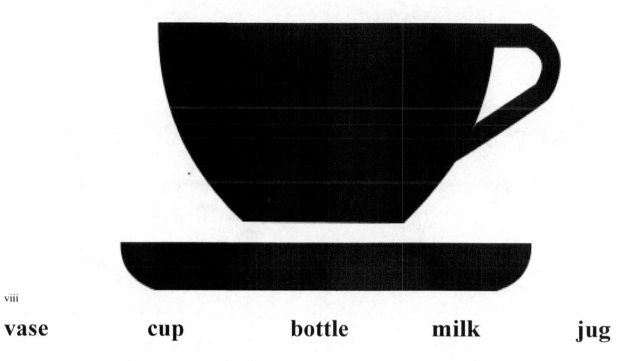

viii

vase   **cup**   **bottle**   **milk**   **jug**

ix

skiing   **sledding**   **jumping**   **flying**   **running**

Matching: Circle the word that matches the picture.

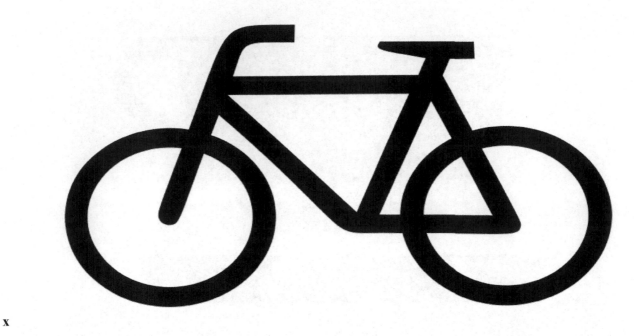

x

skateboard   scooter   unicycle   wagon   bicycle

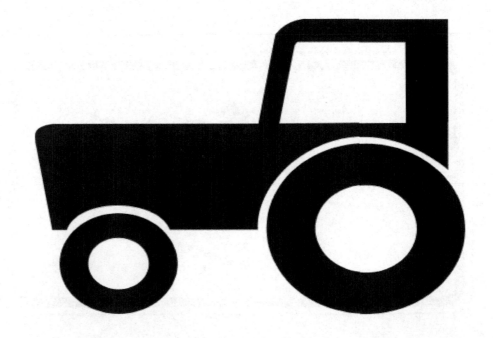

xi

boat   tractor   train   dirt-bike   jet-ski

Matching: Circle the word that matches the picture.

xii

bus   car   skates   jet   motorcycle

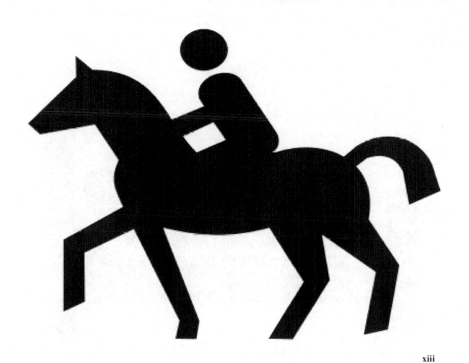

xiii

swimming   jogging   tennis   fishing   horseback riding

Matching: Circle the word that matches the picture.

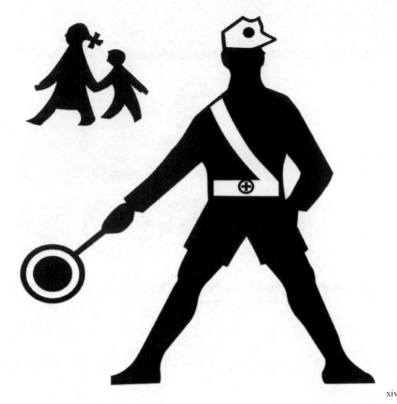

xiv

crossing guard   fireman   janitor   banker   teacher

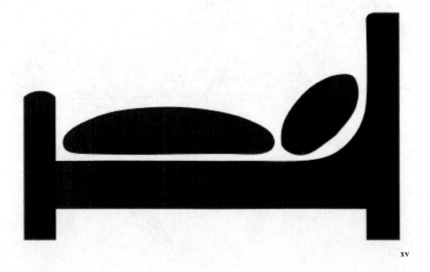

xv

couch   chair   futon   bed   table

Matching: Circle the word that matches the picture.

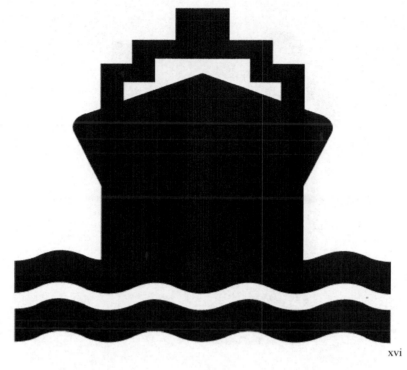

xvi

surfboard   dolphin   ship   sand   whale

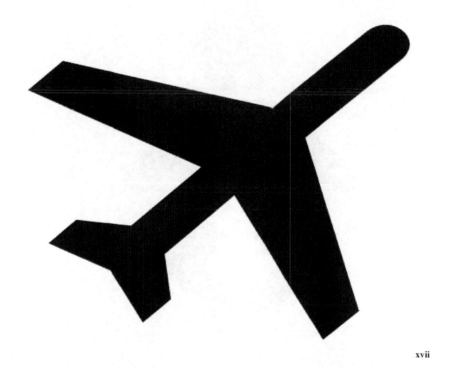

xvii

balloon   blimp   hat   airplane   plug

Matching: Circle the word that matches the picture.

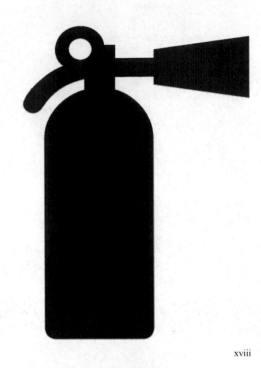

xviii

hose   cup   **fire extinguisher**   sand   water

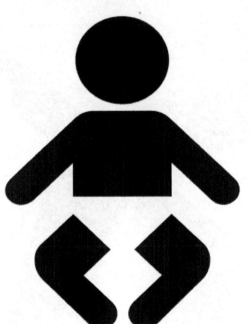

xix

rattle   baby   feet   crib   blanket

Matching: Circle the word that matches the picture.

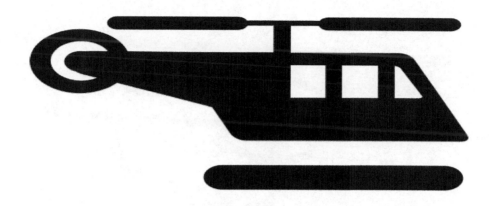

xx

jet ski   blimp   hanger   helicopter   hair

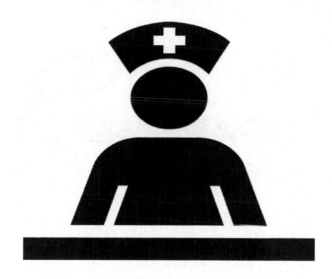

xxi

banker   waitress   nurse   teller   driver

Matching: Circle the word that matches the picture.

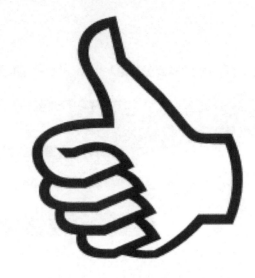

xxii

no   peace   thumbs up   go away   bad

xxiii

cigarette   pipe   glasses   fire   pencil

Matching: Match the word to the symbol.

Point to the snowflake.

 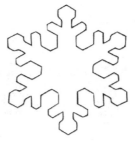  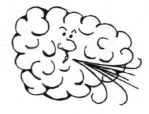

Point to the Escalator.

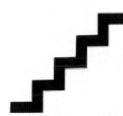   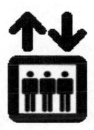

Point to the arrow that points down and to the left.

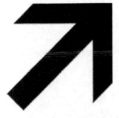  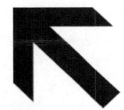 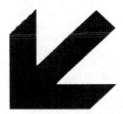

Point to the no smoking sign.

   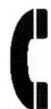

Matching: Match the word to the symbol.

Point to the barber shop for men.

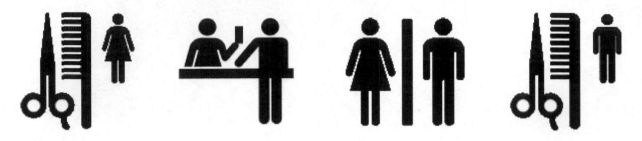

Point to the man throwing away trash.

Point to the crime.

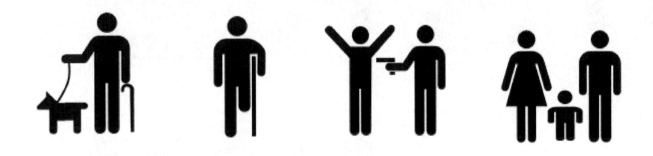

Point to the fork and knife.

Matching: Match the word to the image.

Point to the wolf.

 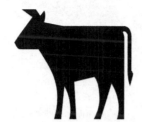 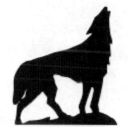 

Point to the snake.

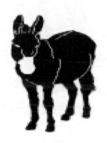 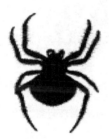 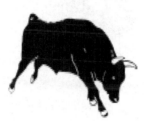 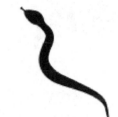

Point to the goat.

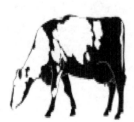 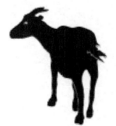 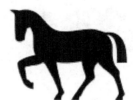 

Point to the dog.

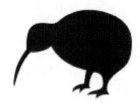 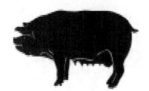 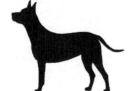 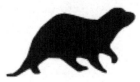

Matching: Match the word to the image.

Point to the cat.

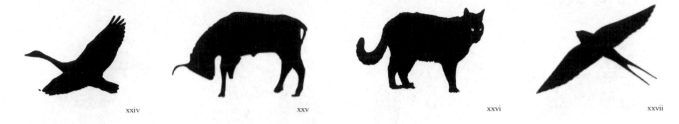

xxiv xxv xxvi xxvii

Point to the dragon.

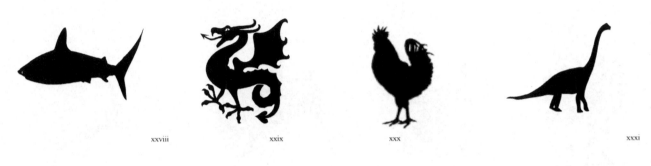

xxviii xxix xxx xxxi

Point to the forest.

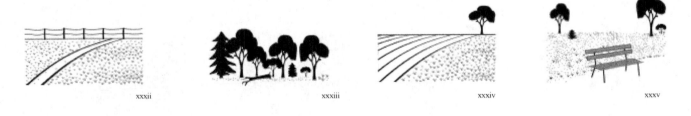

xxxii xxxiii xxxiv xxxv

Point to the lake.

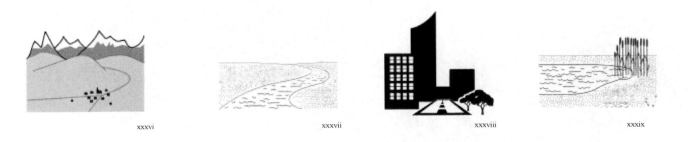

xxxvi xxxvii xxxviii xxxix

Matching: Actions to Pictures.

Point to the person kicking.

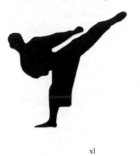 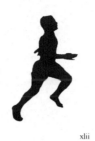 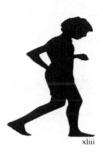

| xl | xli | xlii | xliii |

Point to the person squatting.

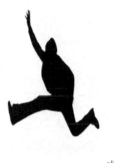 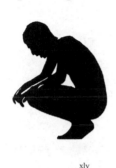 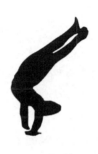 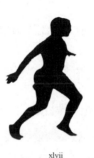

| xliv | xlv | xlvi | xlvii |

Point to the person hanging in the air.

  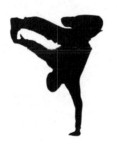 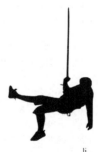

| xlviii | xlix | l | li |

Point to the person playing the guitar.

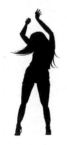 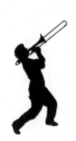 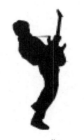 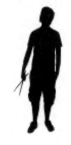

| lii | liii | liv | lv |

Yes/No Questions
Personal

1.	Do you have curly hair?	YES	NO
2.	Do you have brown eyes?	YES	NO
3.	Are you a teenager?	YES	NO
4.	Are you married?	YES	NO
5.	Do you have children?	YES	NO
6.	Are you divorced?	YES	NO
7.	Are you from Chicago?	YES	NO
8.	Are you a teacher?	YES	NO
9.	Do you speak English?	YES	NO
10.	Can you play a musical instrument?	YES	NO
11.	Are you over 5 feet tall?	YES	NO
12.	Do you have grandchildren?	YES	NO
13.	Do you have gray hair?	YES	NO
14.	Do you wear glasses?	YES	NO
15.	Do you have a beard?	YES	NO
16.	Are you retired?	YES	NO
17.	Do you have any pets?	YES	NO
18.	Are you wearing shoes?	YES	NO
19.	Do you wear dentures?	YES	NO
20.	Are your nails painted?	YES	NO

Yes/No Questions
Personal

1. Are you tall?	YES	NO
2. Are you skinny?	YES	NO
3. Is your shoe size larger than size 10?	YES	NO
4. Are you a brunette?	YES	NO
5. Are you bald?	YES	NO
6. Do you have a mustache?	YES	NO
7. Are you bilingual?	YES	NO
8. Are you a meteorologist?	YES	NO
9. Do you live in a city?	YES	NO
10. Do you have children?	YES	NO
11. Do you have any tattoos?	YES	NO
12. Are your ears pierced?	YES	NO
13. Do you have any cavities?	YES	NO
14. Do you have long hair?	YES	NO
15. Do you have cats?	YES	NO
16. Do you have any allergies?	YES	NO
17. Do you have a maid?	YES	NO
18. Are you psychic?	YES	NO
19. Are you wearing a watch?	YES	NO
20. Do you have a pacemaker?	YES	NO

Yes/No Questions
Personal

1. Do you like to watch golf on TV?   YES   NO

2. Do you like seafood?   YES   NO

3. Have you been to Hawaii?   YES   NO

4. Can you swim?   YES   NO

5. Do you like dogs?   YES   NO

6. Have you ever been skiing?   YES   NO

7. Do you like to dance?   YES   NO

8. Do you like to drink beer?   YES   NO

9. Have you been to Rome?   YES   NO

10. Have you ever crocheted a blanket?   YES   NO

11. Do you like horror movies?   YES   NO

12. Do you like sushi?   YES   NO

13. Do you drink coffee?   YES   NO

14. Do you smoke?   YES   NO

15. Have you seen a Broadway play?   YES   NO

16. Do you like to watch Fox News?   YES   NO

17. Are you a Libertarian?   YES   NO

18. Do you believe in ghosts?   YES   NO

19. Do you have a solar powered car?   YES   NO

20. Have you been camping?   YES   NO

Yes/No Questions
Environment

1. Are you in the hospital?	YES	NO
2. Are you lying down?	YES	NO
3. Are you in an office?	YES	NO
4. Are we in Canada?	YES	NO
5. Is there a window in this room?	YES	NO
6. Does this room have two doors?	YES	NO
7. Are you in a wheelchair?	YES	NO
8. Are we in the United States?	YES	NO
9. Is it night time?	YES	NO
10. Have you had breakfast?	YES	NO
11. Are we on the East Coast?	YES	NO
12. Are you wearing your clothes?	YES	NO
13. Did you have a stroke?	YES	NO
14. Are the walls pink?	YES	NO
15. Does the window have curtains?	YES	NO
16. Are we in a church?	YES	NO
17. Are the lights on?	YES	NO
18. Are there children in here?	YES	NO
19. Are you in speech therapy?	YES	NO
20. Are there two chairs in here?	YES	NO

Yes/No Questions
Historical

1. Did Japan attack Pearl Harbor?   YES   NO

2. Did Christopher Columbus "discover" America?   YES   NO

3. Did Picasso paint the Sistine Chapel ceiling?   YES   NO

4. Was the Revolutionary War fought against Spain?   YES   NO

5. Did an onion famine occur in Ireland in the 1840s?   YES   NO

6. Did Hitler lead Germany in an attack against France? YES   NO

7. Did the Titanic sink?   YES   NO

8. Did Magellan sail around the world?   YES   NO

9. Was Charles Lindbergh a pilot?   YES   NO

10. Was the Luftwaffe a fleet of English ships?   YES   NO

11. Was Prohibition the ban of cigarettes in the 1920s?   YES   NO

12. Was Chamberlain an English Prime Minister?   YES   NO

13. Did FDR create the New Deal?   YES   NO

14. Was Nixon president in the 1990s?   YES   NO

15. Was Obama the U.S.'s first Hispanic president?   YES   NO

16. Was Ghengis Khan a human rights activist?   YES   NO

17. Was Marie Curie a famous scientist?   YES   NO

18. Did Gandhi advocate for war in India?   YES   NO

19. Did Einstein create the theory of relativity?   YES   NO

20. Were there 17 original colonies in North America?   YES   NO

Yes/No Questions
Cultural

1. Was Paul McCartney the lead singer of the Beatles?   YES   NO

2. Was John Lennon the drummer for the Beatles?   YES   NO

3. Is Elvis Presley alive?   YES   NO

4. Was the Sound of Music set in France?   YES   NO

5. Did Dorothy from the *Wizard of Oz* befriend a lion?   YES   NO

6. Was *Gone with the Wind* set in the American South?   YES   NO

7. Was Betty Davis know for her large ears?   YES   NO

8. Were the Rolling Stones a rock band?   YES   NO

9. Is *Fiddler on the Roof* a famous musical?   YES   NO

10. Did Charles Dickens write the *Christmas Carol*?   YES   NO

11. Did people wear bell bottom pants in the 1920s?   YES   NO

12. Werc the Three Stooges a comedy team?   YES   NO

13. Did Shirley Temple start her career as an adult?   YES   NO

14. Is *Miracle on 34th Street* a war film?   YES   NO

15. Was Leonard Bernstein a famous composer?   YES   NO

16. Was Mozart a movie star?   YES   NO

17. Is the novel/movie *War of the Worlds* a true story?   YES   NO

18. Was Julia Child a famous chef?   YES   NO

19. Was Michael Jackson known as the "King of Jazz"?   YES   NO

20. Are baby boomers children born after WWII?   YES   NO

Yes/No Questions
Seasonal

1. Does Summer come before spring?   YES   NO

2. Is Valentine's Day in March?   YES   NO

3. Do we rake leaves in autumn?   YES   NO

4. Is your birthday in May?   YES   NO

5. Do children go back to school in June?   YES   NO

6. Does it snow in February?   YES   NO

7. Is Thanksgiving in October?   YES   NO

8. Do children go trick-or-treating in April?   YES   NO

9. Do April showers bring May flowers?   YES   NO

10. Do people like to swim in the ocean in the summer?   YES   NO

11. Do flowers bloom in below freezing temperatures?   YES   NO

12. Are elections held in November?   YES   NO

13. Is Father's Day in June?   YES   NO

14. Do animals hibernate in spring?   YES   NO

15. Is hurricane season in the summer?   YES   NO

16. Do we build snowmen in the winter?   YES   NO

17. Is New Year's Day in December?   YES   NO

18. Is Independence Day in July?   YES   NO

19. Is Christmas always on December 25th?   YES   NO

20. Is Easter in the summer?   YES   NO

Yes/No Questions
Household

1. Does a kitchen have a refrigerator?   YES   NO

2. Are knives use for stirring?   YES   NO

3. Do wet clothes go in the washing machine?   YES   NO

4. Do you put a dryer sheet in the washing machine?   YES   NO

5. Can you microwave metal?   YES   NO

6. Do you dry your hair before you wash it?   YES   NO

7. Do you floss your teeth with a toothbrush?   YES   NO

8. Do you use bleach to darken your hair?   YES   NO

9. Do you preheat the oven before baking?   YES   NO

10. Do you put your socks on before your shoes?   YES   NO

11. Should you touch wet paint?   YES   NO

12. Do you wear reading glasses if you are farsighted?   YES   NO

13. Do you keep milk in the pantry?   YES   NO

14. Do pillows go under the bed?   YES   NO

15. Do you keep ice cream in the refrigerator?   YES   NO

16. Do you flush the toilet after you use it?   YES   NO

17. Do you use aftershave before you shave?   YES   NO

18. Do you steam clean a dirty carpet?   YES   NO

19. Do you mow hardwood floors?   YES   NO

20. Do you put on pajamas when you wake up?   YES   NO

Yes/No Questions
Before and After

1. Do you boil water before you put in a tea bag? YES NO

2. Do you brush your hair before you take a shower? YES NO

3. Do you clean up the paper before you open a present? YES NO

4. Do you soak a stain in detergent before you wash it? YES NO

5. Do you sweep the floor before you mop it? YES NO

6. Do you wash your hands after you use the restroom? YES NO

7. Do you buy popcorn when you leave a movie theater? YES NO

8. Do you curl your hair after you straighten it? YES NO

9. Do you eat garlic before you go to the dentist? YES NO

10. Do you buy a Christmas tree after New Year's Day YES NO

11. Do you light a match before you start a fire? YES NO

12. Do you use a dust pan before you start sweeping? YES NO

13. Do you park your car before you go into a store? YES NO

14. Do you put mayonnaise on bread before you toast it? YES NO

15. Do you use your turn signal before you turn? YES NO

16. Do you order appetizers after the main course? YES NO

17. Can you vote after election day? YES NO

18. Do you test drive a car after you buy it? YES NO

19. Do you make reservations at a restaurant after you eat? YES NO

20. Do you use a vacuum after you spill cereal? YES NO

Yes/No Questions
Meals

1.	Do you put cream on your cereal?	YES	NO
2.	Do you drink coffee at bedtime?	YES	NO
3.	Is brunch a combination of lunch and breakfast?	YES	NO
4.	Is caviar quail eggs?	YES	NO
5.	Is escargot snails?	YES	NO
6.	Do you serve dessert first?	YES	NO
7.	Can you grill salmon?	YES	NO
8.	Can you fry a turkey?	YES	NO
9.	Is a Shirley Temple an alcoholic drink?	YES	NO
10.	Does stuffing go on the outside of a turkey?	YES	NO
11.	If you have a nut allergy, can you eat peanut butter?	YES	NO
12.	Would a vegetarian eat a hot dog?	YES	NO
13.	Is veal a type of pork?	YES	NO
14.	Is coleslaw made of cabbage?	YES	NO
15.	Is fine dining inexpensive?	YES	NO
16.	Does continental sometimes refer to breakfast?	YES	NO
17.	Does a waiter take your order at a picnic?	YES	NO
18.	Does sushi have raw fish in it?	YES	NO
19.	Is 5% considered a good tip for a waiter?	YES	NO
20.	Can you wear pajamas if you order room service?	YES	NO

Yes/No Questions
Safety

1. Should you blow dry your hair while taking a bath?   YES   NO

2. Should you lock the breaks on a wheelchair to sit down? YES   NO

3. Should you run on a wet floor?   YES   NO

4. Should you always wear a seat belt?   YES   NO

5. Should your doors be unlocked when you leave home?   YES   NO

6. Should you drive after you take a sleeping pill?   YES   NO

7. Should you wash a cut before you put on a band aid?   YES   NO

8. Should you take a pill you find on the floor?   YES   NO

9. Should you call for a nurse if you need help getting up?   YES   NO

10. Should you lock your walker before you stand up?   YES   NO

11. Should you reach back and hold the chair before you sit? YES   NO

12. Should you eat lying down in bed?   YES   NO

13. Should you call 411 in an emergency?   YES   NO

14. Should you drive fast on icy roads?   YES   NO

15. Should you take small bites and eat slowly?   YES   NO

16. Should you leave the oven on when you are out?   YES   NO

17. Should you keep emergency contact info with you?   YES   NO

18. Should you wash your hands before you eat?   YES   NO

19. Is it a good idea to have safety bars in a shower?   YES   NO

20. Should you stand on a chair with wheels?   YES   NO

Yes/No Questions
Real or Not

1.	Is a unicorn real?	YES	NO
2.	Is a hedgehog real?	YES	NO
3.	Is a dinosaur real?	YES	NO
4.	Is a griffon real?	YES	NO
5.	Is the Easter Bunny real?	YES	NO
6.	Is a psychiatrist real?	YES	NO
7.	Is a vampire real?	YES	NO
8.	Is an obstetrician real?	YES	NO
9.	Is an elf real?	YES	NO
10.	Is a mole real?	YES	NO
11.	Is a kangaroo real?	YES	NO
12.	Is a polar bear real?	YES	NO
13.	Is a dragon real?	YES	NO
14.	Is a princess real?	YES	NO
15.	Is a mermaid real?	YES	NO
16.	Is a dolphin real?	YES	NO
17.	Is Medusa real?	YES	NO
18.	Is a minotaur real?	YES	NO
19.	Is a pekingese real?	YES	NO
20.	Is a tiger real?	YES	NO

Yes/No Questions
Geography

1. Is Canada south of the United States of America?   YES   NO

2. Is California on the Atlantic Ocean?   YES   NO

3. Is Hawaii in the Pacific Ocean?   YES   NO

4. Is Brazil in North America?   YES   NO

5. Is New Zealand near Australia?   YES   NO

6. Is London the capital of England?   YES   NO

7. Is the Eiffel Tower in Paris?   YES   NO

8. Are the ancient pyramids in Rome?   YES   NO

9. Is Sicily in the Mediterranean Sea?   YES   NO

10. Is Nigeria in Africa?   YES   NO

11. Is the Nile River in Canada?   YES   NO

12. Is Germany in Europe?   YES   NO

13. Does North Korea border China?   YES   NO

14. Is Sydney a city in Australia?   YES   NO

15. Is Mexico north of the United States of America?   YES   NO

16. Is Panama in Central America?   YES   NO

17. Is Moscow the capital of China?   YES   NO

18. Is Sweden part of the United Kingdom?   YES   NO

19. Does Egypt border the Mediterranean Sea?   YES   NO

20. Is Thailand in Asia?   YES   NO

Yes/No Questions
U.S.A. Geography

1.	Does Texas border Mexico?	YES	NO
2.	Is Florida on the Gulf of Mexico?	YES	NO
3.	Does the Mississippi River run east to west?	YES	NO
4.	Is North Dakota above South Dakota?	YES	NO
5.	Is Georgia south of Pennsylvania?	YES	NO
6.	Is Puerto Rico a U.S. State?	YES	NO
7.	Does Alaska border Washington State?	YES	NO
8.	Is the District of Columbia a State?	YES	NO
9.	Does Arizona border Canada?	YES	NO
10.	Is New York City on an island?	YES	NO
11.	Is Philadelphia in New Jersey?	YES	NO
12.	Is San Francisco in California?	YES	NO
13.	Is Virginia a Mid-West State?	YES	NO
14.	Are there ten Great Lakes?	YES	NO
15.	Does Oregon border California?	YES	NO
16.	Is Salt Lake City in Utah?	YES	NO
17.	Is Arkansas on the East Coast?	YES	NO
18.	Is Mississippi in the South?	YES	NO
19.	Is Montana on the Gulf of Mexico?	YES	NO
20.	Is Delaware on the Atlantic Ocean?	YES	NO

Yes/No Questions Inferences

1. He put on a coat and grabbed an umbrella.

   Was it snowing?   YES   NO

2. She called her doctor and needed to be seen as soon as possible.

   Was she sick?   YES   NO

3. He is lactose intolerant.

   Can he have ice cream?   YES   NO

4. The children woke up and ran downstairs to find presents under the tree.

   Was it Easter?   YES   NO

5. He sat on the couch, picked up the remote and grabbed a bag of chips.

   Was he going to make a phone call?   YES   NO

6. She wrote down a list of ingredients: chocolate chips, sugar, flour, baking
   soda, butter, and vanilla.

   Was she going to bake cookies?   YES   NO

7. He got an ice pack, took an Advil and rubbed his knee and laid down.

   Was he feeling well?   YES   NO

8. He swatted the air and starting swinging at the buzzing sound.

   Was a dog bothering him?   YES   NO

9. She put artificial sweeteners in her coffee, and checked her blood sugar.

   Was she diabetic?   YES   NO

10. The trash cans were crooked, turned on their side and had their lids open.

    Did the garbage truck already come?   YES   NO

Yes/No Questions Inferences

1. At the vineyard, they took off their shoes and began to stomp in a large barrel.

   - Were they crushing grapes? YES NO

2. There was a memorial special to remember a movie star.

   -Is the movie star alive? YES NO

3. I put on my running shoes, jacket, grabbed my music and water.

   -Was I going for a jog? YES NO

4. The puppy was inside for 6 hours. When I returned, there was an unpleasant odor.

   -Did the puppy have an accident inside the house? YES NO

5. He ate a peanut butter sandwich for the first time and began to swell up.

   -Could he have a nut allergy? YES NO

6. The man walked up to the gas station with a gas can and filled it up. He asked

   another patron for a ride to his car, 2 miles away.

   -Did his car have a full tank of gas? YES NO

7. That night the 8 year old put a tooth under her pillow and was very excited.

   -Was Santa going to come? Yes NO

8. The bell rang and the girl began to run to her class.

   - Was she early? YES NO

9. The restaurant didn't have lids on kids' cups. The Mom got up from the table and

   asked the waitress for a lot of paper towels.

   - Did her kids spill? YES NO

10. At the checkout counter, he began to pat his pockets and look in his jacket.

    - Was he looking for his wallet? YES NO

Yes/No Definitions

1. Is a carrot a vegetable that grows underground?   YES   NO

2. Is a hubcap a piece of jewelry?   YES   NO

3. Is a rubber band used as an adhesive?   YES   NO

4. Will a twin bed comfortably fit two people?   YES   NO

5. Is a dry erase marker used on a white board?   YES   NO

6. Is a microphone a miniature phone?   YES   NO

7. Is pizza a type of Italian food?   YES   NO

8. Is a caterpillar a young butterfly?   YES   NO

9. Is Pluto considered to be a planet?   YES   NO

10. Is a hamster a rat?   YES   NO

11. Will a permanent tattoo wash off with soap?   YES   NO

12. Is a cub a baby bear?   YES   NO

13. Do Eskimos live in the desert?   YES   NO

14. Are galoshes waterproof?   YES   NO

15. Can a phone take a picture?   YES   NO

16. Do turtles have a soft shell?   YES   NO

17. Do jellyfish sting?   YES   NO

18. Are doughnuts a health food?   YES   NO

19. Do mice catch cats?   YES   NO

20. Are engagement rings typically rubies?   YES   NO

Yes/No Definitions (locations)

1. Do you keep a rolling pin in the bathroom?	YES	NO
2. Do you keep a toolbox in the garage?	YES	NO
3. Do you store old clothes in the attic?	YES	NO
4. Do you put cinnamon in the medicine cabinet?	YES	NO
5. Do you put silverware in a toy box?	YES	NO
6. Do you put makeup in the refrigerator?	YES	NO
7. Does a computer go in the bathroom?	YES	NO
8. Do you hang a calendar on the wall?	YES	NO
9. Do you put receipts in a frame?	YES	NO
10. Do you put books on a bookshelf?	YES	NO
11. Do you keep jewelry and passports in a safe?	YES	NO
12. Do you keep pajamas in your purse?	YES	NO
13. Does a star go at the base of a Christmas tree?	YES	NO
14. Could you keep a stapler in a desk drawer?	YES	NO
15. Do you put outgoing mail in the mailbox?	YES	NO
16. Do you find a water heater in a dining room?	YES	NO
17. Does a washer/dryer go in a laundry room?	YES	NO
18. Do bikes go in a coat closet?	YES	NO
19. Do spoons go in a kitchen drawer?	YES	NO
20. Do sheets and towels go in a hall closet?	YES	NO

Yes/No Questions

1. Is your nose an internal organ?   YES   NO

2. Is a King an elected official?   YES   NO

3. Should you fly a flag at night?   YES   NO

4. Is Yellowstone a National Park?   YES   NO

5. Do children ride to school on a Greyhound bus?   YES   NO

6. Is a limousine a form of public transportation?   YES   NO

7. Is first class cheaper than coach?   YES   NO

8. Do you use a microscope to look at the stars?   YES   NO

9. Does a speedometer tell you how fast you are driving?   YES   NO

10. Do you use a thermometer to measure medicine?   YES   NO

11. Do you stand at a podium in a movie theater?   YES   NO

12. Do you add ice to raise the temperature?   YES   NO

13. If you dive underwater, will your hair get wet?   YES   NO

14. Do kangaroos carry their baby in a pouch?   YES   NO

15. Do you use a tissue when you are sick?   YES   NO

16. Does a carpenter set up electrical wires?   YES   NO

17. Does a pediatrician treat geriatric patients?   YES   NO

18. Do you cough with your nose?   YES   NO

19. Can you take a bath in a shower stall?   YES   NO

20. Can you cut down trees with scissors?   YES   NO

Yes/No Questions

1. Is baseball a sport?   YES   NO

2. Do elephants live on a farm?   YES   NO

3. Is tea a beverage?   YES   NO

4. Are nachos a dessert?   YES   NO

5. Is lemonade a soda?   YES   NO

6. Is swimming an exercise?   YES   NO

7. Is a cardiologist a doctor?   YES   NO

8. Is cauliflower a vegetables?   YES   NO

9. Is a jacket an undergarment?   YES   NO

10. Are eggs a breakfast food?   YES   NO

11. Is Chevrolet a type of car?   YES   NO

12. Is a marigold a type of tree?   YES   NO

13. Is vanilla an ice cream flavor?   YES   NO

14. Is a visor a type of footwear?   YES   NO

15. Do monkeys live in the jungle?   YES   NO

16. Is a pencil a school supply?   YES   NO

17. Is a guitar a musical instrument?   YES   NO

18. Do you watch movies in the garage?   YES   NO

19. Is a broom a cleaning tool?   YES   NO

20. Is a necklace a dog toy?   YES   NO

When Questions

1. When is Thanksgiving?

November   March   December   April

2. When is Labor Day?

April   September   January   May

3. When is Valentine's Day?

February   April   May   June

4. When is Pearl Harbor Day?

August   October   September   December

5. When is Mother's Day?

May   June   August   April

6. When is Father's Day?

May   June   April   October

7. When is Christmas?

January   March   May   December

8. When is New Year's Day?

December   February   January   March

9. When is Independence Day?

June   July   August   September

10. When is Memorial Day?

March   September   October   May

When Questions

1. When do you shovel snow?

   Autumn   Winter   Spring   Summer

2. When was World War II?

   1920s   1960s   1930s   1940s

3. When was the American Civil War?

   1960s   1740s   1860s   1850s

4. When was the World Trade Center attacked in New York City?

   2011   1911   2001   1991

5. When is the evening news on TV?

   2:00 pm   6:00 am   6:00 pm   8:00 pm

6. When do people like to go to the beach?

   Fall   Winter   Summer   Spring

7. When do people usually drink wine?

   Breakfast   5:00 am   Driving   Dinner

8. When do you have lunch?

   Midday   Nighttime   Evening   Morning

9. When was George Washington president of the United States?

   1750s   1850s   1790s   1990s

10. When do you go to the dentist?

    Weekly   Daily   Monthly   Bi-annually

Who Questions

1. Who puts out fires?

   Policeman   Plumber   Electrician   Fireman

2. Who stops crime?

   Toll Taker   Nurse   Undertaker   Policeman

3. Who is in jail?

   Santa   Criminals   Ice Skaters   Artists

4. Who installs light fixtures?

   Landscaper   Electrician   Doctor   Archeologist

5. Who builds houses?

   Teacher   Contractor   Welder   Mail Carrier

6. Who catalogs books?

   Nurse   Engineer   Librarian   Brick Layer

7. Who checks your eyes?

   Dermatologist   Ophthalmologist   Gynecologist   Podiatrist

8. Who makes your food at a restaurant?

   Hostess   Waitress   Cook   Delivery Man

9. Who writes news stories?

   Anchorman   Journalist   Singer   Author

10. Who performs on Broadway?

    Actors   Salesmen   Cashier   Street Performers

Who Questions

1. Who is Dolly Parton?

    Politician   Scientist   Country Music Star   Housewife

2. Who is Queen Elizabeth II?

    Queen of England   Queen of France   Queen of Belgium   Queen of Austria

3. Who is Brad Pitt?

    Author   Senator   Movie Star   CEO

4. Who is Barack Obama?

    Ambassador   President   Philanthropist   Psychologist

5. Who is Nelson Mandela?

    South African President/Activist   Singer   Actor   Rock Star

6. Who is Mahatma Gandhi?

    Inventor   Professor   Athlete   Indian Activist

7. Who is Mother Teresa?

    Charitable Catholic Nun   Nurse   Doctor   Teacher

8. Who is Sonia Sotomayor?

    Comedian   Blues Singer   Supreme Court Justice   Senator

9. Who is Vladimir Putin?

    German President   Russian President King of Austria   Australian President

10. Who is Vivian Lee?

    Artist   Actress   Philanthropist   Educator

Where Questions

1. Where do you keep your medication?

   Kitchen Drawer   Shed   Desk   Medicine Cabinet

2. Where do you keep your winter coats?

   Crawl Space   Attic   Coat Closet   Bathroom

3. Where do you keep pots and pans

   Kitchen Cabinet   Refrigerator   Garage   Basement

4. Where do you keep a shovel?

   Pantry   Dining Room   Living Room   Garage

5. Where do you keep socks?

   Refrigerator   Desk   Closet   Dresser Drawer

6. Where do you keep china place settings?

   Swing   Deck   Cabinet   Oven

7. Where is the fireplace?

   Bathroom   Crawlspace   Attic   Living Room

8. Where is a swimming pool typically?

   Roof   Basement   Backyard   Front Yard

9. Where would you find a picnic table?

   Formal Dining Room   Bathroom   Hallway   Park

10. Where do you keep the salt and pepper shakers?

   Floor   Hall Closet   Kitchen Table   Desk

Where Questions

1. Where is Atlanta?

   Virginia   Ohio   Georgia   South Carolina

2. Where is Chicago?

   Indiana   Michigan   Illinois   Idaho

3. Where is Salt Lake City?

   Arizona   Utah   Oklahoma   New Mexico

4. Where is Los Angeles?

   Oregon   Washington   California   Nevada

5. Where is San Diego?

   Arizona   Florida   Georgia   California

6. Where is Las Vegas?

   California   Arizona   Nevada   Utah

7. Where is Seattle?

   Colorado   Montana   North Dakota   Washington

8. Where is Boston?

   Connecticut   Massachusetts   New York   Vermont

9. Where is New Orleans?

   Mississippi   Florida   Arkansas   Louisiana

10. Where is Miami?

    Florida   California   Cuba   Georgia

What Questions

1. What is a giraffe?

   Chair   Color   Insect   Animal

2. What is a Mercedes?

   Flower   Shampoo   Luxury Car   Tree

3. What is a ring?

   Jewelry   Hat   Tool   Rose

4. What is a dress?

   Food   Weights   Clothing   Tool

5. What is a Beagle?

   Instrument   Cat   Shoe   Dog

6. What is aspirin?

   Candy   Vitamin   Medicine   Drink

7. What is lipstick?

   Lotion   Hair Product   Makeup   Clothing

8. What is a couch?

   TV   Furniture   Fireplace   Armor

9. What is a hammer?

   Rock   Car   Jewel   Tool

10. What is pink?

   Fire   Rainbow   Color   Pants

What Questions: (personal)

1. What is your mother's maiden name?

2. What is your birthstone?

3. What was your profession?

4. What are your parents' names?

5. What are the ages of your children?

6. What do you like better, dogs or cats?

7. What is your nationality?

8. What was your favorite subject in school?

9. What do you prefer, coffee or tea?

10. What do you prefer, beer or wine?

11. What is your political party?

12. What is your religion?

13. What is your spouse's name?

14. What are your hobbies?

15. What is your email address?

16. What is your home address?

17. What is your phone number?

18. What is your favorite TV show?

19. What sports do you like to watch?

20. What is your middle name?

One Step Directions:

1. Tap your knee

2. Touch your nose

3. Put your hand on your hip

4. Run your fingers through your hair

5. Shrug you shoulders

6. Kick your left foot

7. Raise your hand

8. Puff out your stomach

9. Give a thumbs up

10. Pat your back

11. Snap your fingers

12. Point to the floor

13. Point to the ceiling

14. Look out the window

15. Laugh

16. Cross your legs

17. Tap your foot

18. Touch your elbow

19. Make a muscle

20. Tug your ear

One Step Directions:

1. Stick out your tongue

2. Smile

3. Move your tongue from left to right

4. Blink your eyes

5. Frown

6. Purse your lips

7. Touch your upper lip with your tongue

8. Turn your head to the right

9. Look down

10. Sniff

11. Clear your throat

12. Wiggle your nose

13. Squint your eyes

14. Raise your eyebrows

15. Puff out your cheeks

16. Whistle

17. Cough

18. Wink

19. Look up

20. Make a "raspberry"

One Step Directions: Immediate surroundings (skip the ones that do not apply)

1. Point to the bed

2. Point to the TV

3. Point to yourself

4. Point to your feet

5. Point to the ceiling

6. Point to the lamp

7. Point to the dresser

8. Point to the call bell

9. Point to the phone

10. Point to a pen

11. Point to a book

12. Point to a pair of shoes

13. Point to the window

14. Point to your chin

15. Point to a pillow

16. Point to a photograph

17. Point to a blanket

18. Point to a ring

19. Point to your leg

20. Point to your teeth

One Step Directions: Pretend to.....

1. Pretend to open a door

2. Brush your hair

3. Start a car

4. Play tennis

5. Sing opera

6. Put on a hat

7. Ride a bike

8. Salute

9. Pledge allegiance

10. Play a flute

11. Thumb your nose

12. Fly

13. Kick a ball

14. Write a letter

15. Eat a sandwich

16. Lick an ice cream cone

17. Dance

18. Brush your teeth

19. Put on a coat

20. Put on a pair of shoes

One Step Directions: Pretend to....

1. Put on a pair of pants

2. Put on a pair of gloves

3. Take off a ring

4. Use a fork

5. Use a hair dryer

6. Shave

7. Use mouthwash

8. Drink a cup of coffee

9. Make a snowball

10. Paint a picture

11. Water the plants

12. Take a picture

13. Put on glasses

14. Scrub a table

15. Dust a shelf

16. Look through a peep hole

17. Ring the doorbell

18. Sweep the floor

19. Lick a stamp

20. Cut with scissors

One Step Directions: Pretend to....

1. Zip up a coat

2. Read a book

3. Wash your hair

4. Make a bed

5. Do the laundry

6. Turn off a faucet

7. Use a salt shaker

8. Put on lipstick

9. Adjust a hearing aid

10. Take a pill

11. Floss your teeth

12. Clean your ears

13. Vacuum

14. Fold laundry

15. Put on deodorant

16. Turn down the radio

17. Roll up the window

18. Paint your nails

19. Use an eraser

20. Sign your name

One Step Directions: Complex

1. Touch your nose if you are wearing sneakers.

2. Pat your knee if you are a woman.

3. Tug your ear if you are a Republican.

4. Stick out your tongue if you like chocolate.

5. Shrug your shoulders if you wear dentures.

6. Nod your head if you are wearing a ring.

7. Kick your foot if the lights are off.

8. Smile if your shirt has buttons.

9. Tap your toes if you are sitting down.

10. Blink if you are wearing glasses.

11. Cross your legs if you are wearing pants.

12. Raise your hand if you live in the United States of America.

13. Pat your belly if we are on the West Coast.

14. Say "Ah" if you are over 50.

15. Snap your fingers if you are wearing a hat.

16. Pat your knee if you have eaten breakfast today.

17. Say "yoo-hoo" if there are blinds on the window.

18. Stomp if it is nighttime.

19. Wiggle your finger if you can hear music.

20. Whistle if the walls are yellow.

One Step Directions: Complex

1. If Christmas is in July, point to the ceiling.

2. If Reagan was a U.S. President, point to the floor.

3. If Mars is a planet, touch your forehead.

4. If roses are black, put your hand on your hip.

5. If it is a weekday, touch your elbow.

6. If libraries lend books, point to a chair.

7. If fire is cold, wave.

8. If dogs bark, pat your back.

9. If school zone speed limits require you to speed up, give a thumbs up.

10. If french fries are made from potatoes, hold your nose.

11. If Walmart is a small business, blink.

12. If tenors are male singers, make a fist.

13. If jalapenos help stop indigestion, clear your throat.

14. If camouflage helps you stand out, clap.

15. If Labor Day is in September, point to your cheek.

16. If John Wayne was a politician, purse your lips.

17. If mouthwash is kept in bathrooms, look up.

18. If you wear a bathing suit to church, take a deep breath.

19. If you wear boots on the beach, cross your fingers.

20. If turkey is served at Thanksgiving, rub your neck.

One Step Directions: Categories

1. Circle the fruit.

   Square   Yellow   Orange   Broccoli   Ham

2. Put a line under the animal.

   Honey   Book   Tape   Bear   Shoe

3. Put an X through the dessert.

   Cake   Ring   Pink   Bowl   Milk

4. Put a line above the cereal.

   Banana   Chips   Cheerios   Milk   Plate

5. Put a line through the eating utensil.

   Ladle   Fork   Mustard   Ketchup   Wallet

6. Circle the fish.

   Snail   Otter   Turtle   Slug   Salmon

7. Put an X to the right of the flower.

   Ivy   Grass   Rose   Pen   Cinnamon

8. Underline the color.

   Paper   Red   Bottle   Diamond   Crayon

9. Circle the dairy product.

   Cheese   Apple   Salt   Pickle   Chips

10. Underline the piece of furniture.

   Window   Mailbox   Shade   Chair   Curtain

One Step Directions: Categories

1. Put a line through the State.

Newark   France   Maine   Gulf   Seattle

2. Circle the item of clothing.

Envelope   Shirt   Card   Window   Gum

3. Underline the movie.

Honeymooners   Disney   Wizard of Oz   Theater

4. Put a line above the insect.

Camel   Mosquito   Monkey   Polish   Swatter

5. Circle the baby toy.

Scissors   Glue   Bag   Rattle   Sock

6. Underline the Country.

Italy   Bank   Ocean   City   Town

7. Put an X to the right of the Girl's name.

Harry   Frank   Bob   Julie   Walter

8. Put an X to the left of the Boy's name.

Sarah   Edward   Avery   Brooke   Mary

9. Circle the cookie.

Doughnut   Cream-puff   Croissant   Cracker   Macaroon

10. Put a line through the car company.

Gucci   Polo   Whirlpool   Intel   Ford

One Step Directions:

Circle the item that doesn't belong in the category.

1. clog   slipper   boot   sock   glove

2. salt   pepper   thyme   lemon   cinnamon

3. brie   margarine   gorgonzola   cheddar   mozzarella

4. crow   cardinal   chipmunk   bluebird   hummingbird

5. ruby   rock   diamond   emerald   opal

6. ax   arrow   sword   string   gun

7. Godiva   Ghirardelli   Hershey   Ivory   Russell Stover

8. brush   screwdriver   wrench   hammer   ratchet

9. Tylenol   Aspirin   Advil   Motrin   Skittles

10. Macy's   Sears   JCPenny   Belk   Walgreens

11. lion   tiger   hamster   giraffe   hippopotamus

12. shih-tzu   mustang   beagle   pug   bulldog

13. paint   crayons   markers   pencil   knife

14. hat   sunglasses   earrings   socks   scarf

15. Florida   New York   Georgia   Delaware   Chicago

16. red   misty   blue   orange   purple

17. square   circle   diamond   oval   large

18. Italy   Ireland   Australia   Spain   Germany

19. guitar   flute   clarinet   drums   grill

20. flag   shovel   rake   pickax   hoe

One Step Directions:

Circle the item that doesn't belong in the category.

1. Visa   MasterCard   Platinum   Discover   American Express

2. oak   maple   rose   pine   hickory

3. Thailand   England   Germany   France   Italy

4. Ivory   Dove   Hallmark   Suave   Neutrogena

5. Paris   Houston   London   Belfast   Rome

6. salsa   tango   oval   rumba   swing

7. crickets   bird   roach   ladybug   beetle

8. spatula   refrigerator   stove   dishwasher   microwave

9. UPS   Fed Ex   Apple   DHL   USPS

10. Cheerios   Toast   Special K   Total   Raisin Bran

11. watch   ring   earring   necklace   hair tie

12. shrimp   lobster   chicken   clams   oysters

13. May   April   October   September   Friday

14. bumper   tailpipe   engine   shoe   wheel

15. jazz   novel   blues   pop   rap

16. Ohio   Atlanta   Charlotte   Charleston   Miami

17. spoon   fork   lemon   plate   knife

18. tape   lipstick   rouge   foundation   mascara

19. Ford   Chevy   Samsung   GM   Cadillac

20. Ireland   Iraq   Iran   Palestine   Egypt

Two Step Directions:

1. Bark like a dog and sniff.

2. Claw like a tiger and growl.

3. Purr like a cat and pretend to pet one.

4. Twitch your nose like a mouse and look left to right.

5. Make galloping noises and pretend your are holding a horse's reigns.

6. Snort like a pig and then hold your nose.

7. Crow like a rooster and sit up straight.

8. Pant like a dog and pretend to lick your paw.

9. Tweet like a bird and flap your arm(s).

10. Hiss like a snake and wiggle back and forth.

11. Scratch like a monkey and say, "ee ee".

12. Move your hand up like a spider and then have the "spider" fall down.

13. Caw like a crow and look up.

14. Quack like a duck and tap your foot.

15. Make a fish face and move your hand like it is swimming.

16. Stretch your neck up like a giraffe and stick out your tongue.

17. "Ba" like a sheep three times.

18. Say "oo" like a gorilla and pound your chest.

19. Flutter your hand like a butterfly and bat your eyelids.

20. Hop your hand like a grasshopper and then turn your hand over.

Two Step Directions:

1. Wave, then close your eyes.

2. Hold up your pinky finger and pretend to drink tea.

3. Stick out your tongue and say "ah".

4. Touch your elbow, then flap your arms.

5. Nod your head, then say "hello".

6. Touch your knee and kick out your leg.

7. Click you tongue, then smile.

8. Snap your finger, then tug your ear.

9. Brush back your hair, then wink.

10. Shrug your shoulders and laugh.

11. Rock back and forth, then salute.

12. Wiggle your foot and look up.

13. Touch your hip and raise your eyebrows.

14. Raise your hand and say "excuse me".

15. Hold out your hand and say "more please".

16. Make a peace sign and stick out your tongue.

17. Point up and pretend to conduct an orchestra.

18. Rub your chin and look suspicious.

19. Turn your hand palm up and look to the right.

20. Roll you eyes and exhale loudly.

Two Step Directions:

1. Point to the ceiling, then to the floor.

2. Point to a chair, then to the table.

3. Point to your throat, then to the window.

4. Point to the right, then to the left.

5. Point to the door, then to the wall.

6. Point under your chair and then point to a book.

7. Point down, then point up.

8. Point to yourself, then point to me.

9. Point to your right ear, then your left ear.

10. Point to a corner, then point to a picture.

11. Point to your jaw and kick your foot.

12. Point below your left eye and say "me".

13. Point to your bicep muscle and then make a fist.

14. Point to your right hand and then purse your lips.

15. Make the okay sign and say "okay".

16. Make a thumbs down and say "boo".

17. Purse your lips, then smile.

18. Point to your stomach, then point to your armpit.

19. Swat the air and say "go away".

20. Point to the chair and then to the bathroom.

Two Step Directions: Complex

1. Before you count to five, snap.

2. After you nod "yes", say "no".

3. Tap your knee three times and pat the other knee twice.

4. Click your tongue twice, then waggle your finger "no".

5. Before you wave, take a deep breath.

6. Draw a Z in the air and then blink 3 times.

7. After you tap your head twice, bow.

8. Before you look down, hug yourself.

9. Move your hand like a puppet as you count down from 10.

10. Tap your foot with your other foot 3 times with your eyes closed.

11. Before you move your tongue side to side, sniff.

12. Say, "good dog" and pretend to pet it three times.

13. Touch every other knuckle on one hand, then touch your elbow.

14. Before you touch your shin, scratch your head.

15. Put your chin in your hand as you raise up your knee.

16. Before you point to the door, blow two kisses.

17. Pretend to spit and then touch your left ear 6 times.

18. Before you adjust your shirt, sit up straight.

19. Look down and up slowly 5 times as you hum.

20. Before you clear your throat, swallow.

Two Step Directions:

1. Circle all the words that end in "s" and underline the color.

   dogs   red   shoe   window   hiss

2. Put an X through all the "r"s in the words and circle the tree.

   pine   rabbit   branch   car   strap

3. Put a diagonal line through all the meats and circle all the vowels.

   veal   apple   steak   carpet   pork

4. Underline the vacation spots and put an X through the animal.

   coyote   Disney World   Bahamas   Hawaii   Desert

5. Circle all the letter "l"s and draw a line above the shoe.

   color   ballet   last   loafers   bracelet

6. Underline the modes of transportation and put an X above all the letter "m"s.

   motorcycle   bus   marathon   subway   tram

7. Circle the fragile items and underline the durable ones.

   china cup   trunk   safe   icicle   barbell

8. Underline the fast food chains and circle the food item.

   lotion   Wendy's   McDonald's   fries   Arby's

9. Circle the body parts and underline the items of clothing.

   nose   arm   shirt   hat   leg

10. Put an X below the tailgating food and circle the fruit.

    hamburger   coffee   peach   tail   shirt

Three Step Directions:

1. Draw a circle in the air, point up, then touch your nose.

2. Laugh, stick out your tongue, and thumb your nose.

3. Point to the chair, touch your eyebrow with two fingers, and look down.

4. Tap your knee with three fingers, tap your toe twice, and point to the ceiling.

5. Put your hand under your armpit before you look up and down.

6. Hum "Jingle Bells" while you look from left to right.

7. Cross your legs with your hand on your bottom knee, and then kick out.

8. Shrug your right shoulder, put your pinky finger on your ear lobe, and frown.

9. Look behind you, then look at your feet and say, "hey".

10. Put one hand on top of the other, tap your finger three times, and touch your chin.

11. Say your name, point to yourself, and smile.

12. Wave to me, point to me, and then wag your finger at me.

13. Before you make a thumbs down, look at your left shoulder, and purse your lips.

14. Flap your arm like a bird four times, make a fist, and then point to the wall.

15. Pretend to eat, chew, and spit out your food.

16. Look out the window, look at the floor, and then look at the ceiling.

17. Touch above your left eye before you point to your ear with your pinky finger but after you smile at me.

18. Before you close your eyes, wink, and look up.

19. Sigh, show your teeth, and then suck in your cheeks.

20. Move your tongue side to side, after you touch each cheek twice.

Three Step Directions:

1. Smile, laugh, then point to me.

2. Tap your foot, tug your ear, then point to the floor.

3. Touch your elbow, wiggle your nose, and say "hello".

4. Wave, stick out your tongue, then look to the left.

5. Point to the door, pat your tummy, and frown.

6. Make a thumbs up, stick out your leg, and look up.

7. Purse your lips, tap your knee 3 times, then look to the right.

8. Draw a square in the air with your finger, touch your head, and then pat your cheek.

9. Hold up your pinky finger, tap your foot 4 times, then cover your ear.

10. Make a peace sign, pretend to fly, and then touch your neck.

11. Before you say "goodbye", snap your fingers and shake your head "no".

12. After you snap your fingers, count backwards from 5, and then clap.

13. Draw a circle on your knee with your finger, close your eyes, and sniff.

14. Stomp your foot 5 times, wave to yourself, and touch the back of your head.

15. Look down, then look to the right, and then snap 3 times.

16. Before you pretend to tie your shoe, put your palm on your shin and sigh.

17. Frown and clear your throat twice after you stick out your tongue.

18. Before you tap the chair twice, wink 3 times and grumble.

19. Pretend to rock a baby in your arm, hum a lullaby and say "shh".

20. Rock back and forth with two fingers in the air while looking down.

Multiple Step Directions With Objects (Materials: Deck of Cards)

1. Take the top card and put in under the deck.

2. Split the deck in half.

3. Take the top card off the right half and look at it

4. If it is a red card, put it under the left stack of cards.

5. If it is a black card, put it under the right stack of cards.

6. Split the two stacks of cards into a total of four stacks.

7. Pick up a card from a middle stack and put in below the stack on the far left.

8. Pick up a card from the other middle stack and put it on top of the stack on the far right.

9. Turn the top cards over on all four stacks.

10. Put all the black cards under the left stack.

11. Put all the red cards under the right stack.

12. Turn the top cards over on all four stacks.

13. Wink twice if there are any cards with spades.

14. If there are no spades, tug your ear.

15. Touch your nose if there are any cards with hearts.

16. If there are no hearts, stick out your tongue

17. Tap the table 5 times if there are any cards with clubs.

18. If there are no clubs, tap the table 8 times.

19. Touch your neck if there are cards with diamonds.

20. If there are no diamonds, shake your head "no" twice and "yes" once.

Multiple Step Directions With Objects (Materials: straw, cup, glove, pen)

1. Put the straw, cup, glove and pen in a row in that order from left to right.

2. Put the pen in the cup.

3. Fold down the middle finger of the glove.

4. Put the straw inside the glove.

5. Put the pen on top of the cup lengthwise pointing to you.

6. Take the pen off of the cup and turn the cup over.

7. Take the straw out of the glove and form an X with the pen.

8. Turn down the pinky finger and the thumb of the glove.

9. Put the cup on the table between you and the glove.

10. Put the glove in the cup and place it to the right of the X.

11. Make the straw and the pen into a T shape.

12. Put the cup above the T and the glove below the T.

13. Put the glove to the right of the T and fold down all the fingers except the pointer.

14. Make the straw and the pen into an L with the pen at the bottom.

15. Lay the pen on the pointer finger of the glove.

16. Put the cup upside down below the glove.

17. Fold the pinky finger of the glove up and lay the straw on it.

18. Put the pen and the straw inside the cup.

19. Take the pen out and place it to the left of the cup.

20. Take the straw out and place it above the glove.

Multiple Step Directions With Objects
(Materials: piece of paper, paper clip, sticky note, and cone)

1. Lie the cone on its side and put the sticky note on it.

2. Put the paper clip under the cone.

3. Put the sticky note on the piece of paper and turn them over.

4. Take the paper clip and put it on top of the paper and place the cone upright.

5. Put the paper clip on the right side of the cone.

6. Put the sticky note under the cone.

7. Put the piece of paper on top of the cone.

8. Pick up the paper clip and move it in the air clockwise around the cone twice.

9. Move the paper clip to the left side of the cone.

10. Take the piece of paper off the cone and put it on the opposite side of the paper clip.

11. Turn the cone over and take out the sticky note.

12. Hold the sticky note up in the air and point it towards the direction of the door.

13. Put the sticky note on the bottom right corner of the piece of paper.

14. Fold the piece of paper in half and place it on your lap.

15. Put the paper clip inside the cone.

16. Take the piece of paper off your lap, unfold it, and move the sticky note to the middle.

17. Take the paper clip out of the cone and put it on top of the sticky note.

18. Put the cone on the top right corner of the piece of paper.

19. Put the paper clip under the cone.

20. Put the sticky note on the back of the cone and then rotate it towards yourself.

Multiple Step Directions With Objects
(Materials: sugar pack, sweetener, fork, and napkin)

1. Line the sugar pack, sweetener, fork and napkin up left to right.

2. Place the fork to the right of the napkin.

3. Put the sugar on top of the sweetener and then put them both on the napkin.

4. Put the fork above the napkin with the prongs facing to the right.

5. Put the sweetener under the fork.

6. Put the sugar pack on the prongs of the fork.

7. Fold the napkin in half and put it to the left of the fork.

8. Place the sugar packet inside the napkin.

9. Put the fork on top of the napkin.

10. Move the sweetener packet to the left side of the napkin and flip it over.

11. Tap the fork three times and place it below the folded napkin pointing at you.

12. Open up the napkin, take out the sugar and put it under the sweetener packet.

13. If the sweetener packet is blue, touch your ear twice and blink three times.

14. If the sweetener packet is pink, tap your foot and stick out your tongue.

15. Move the sweetener packet above the napkin on the table.

16. Flip the sugar packet over and move the fork below the sugar.

17. Put the fork on the napkin. Place the sugar on the left and the sweetener on the right.

18. Switch the places of the sweetener and sugar and put the fork under the napkin.

19. Put the napkin on your lap.

20. Put the sweetener packet and the sugar packet between the prongs of the fork.

Multiple Directions with Images

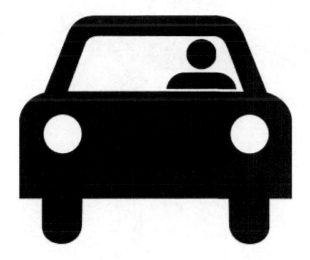

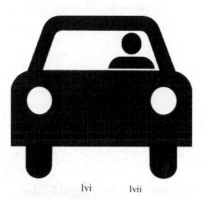

lvi   lvii

1. Put an X above the light bulb.

2. Draw a line from the small car to the trees.

3. Circle the light bulb and put a check mark below the larger car.

4. Draw an arrow pointing to the pine tree.

5. Draw a smiley face on the light bulb.

Multiple Step Directions with Images

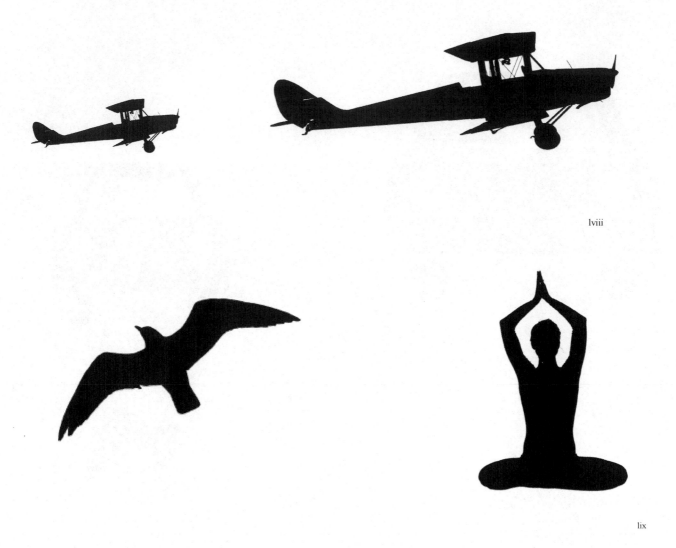

lviii

lix

1. On the bottom right corner of each picture, write a number. Number the bird 1, the woman doing yoga 2, the large plane 3 and the small plane 4.

2. Draw a line from the bird to the large plane and then to the woman.

3. Circle the small plane twice.

4. Draw an X through the woman and draw a circle below the small plane.

5. Make 2 dots under the small plane and 4 dots above the large plane.

Multiple Step Directions with Images

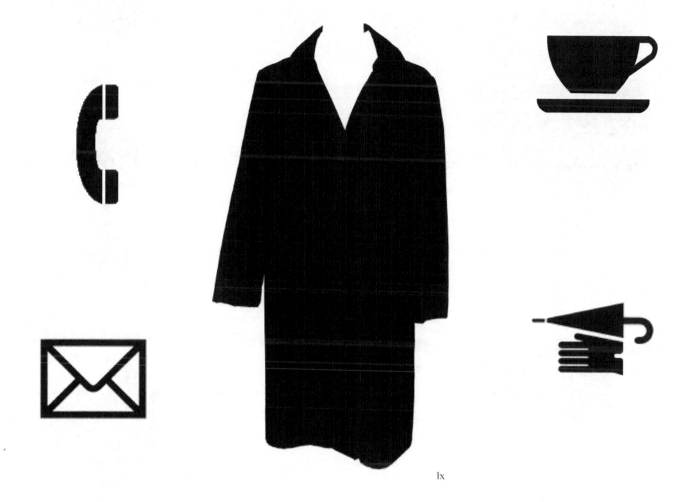

lx

1. Draw a line from the phone, around the envelope, under the coat and to the glove.

2. Draw a line from the cup, through the umbrella and glove, up over the coat and to the phone.

3. Draw a star above the envelope, under the cup and to the right of the glove.

4. Circle the three objects you pick up and bring to your mouth.

5. Draw a line from the umbrella to the phone but do not go through the coat.

Multiple Step Directions with Images

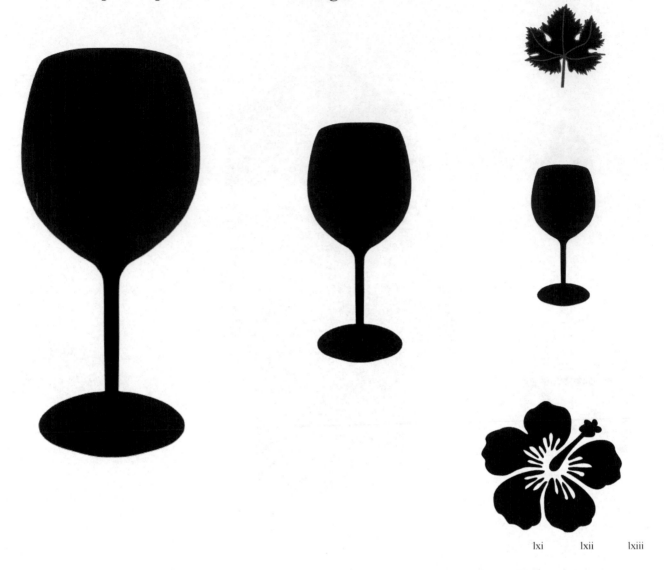

1. Put a check mark to the left of the medium wine glass and to the right of the smallest wine glass.

2. Draw a circle, square and rectangle under the largest wine glass.

3. Draw a line from the flower to the largest wine glass and a line from the smallest wine glass to the leaf.

4. Draw a line from the leaf to every image except the medium sized wine glass.

5. Draw a line from the largest wine glass to the flower and leaf.

Multiple Step Directions with Images

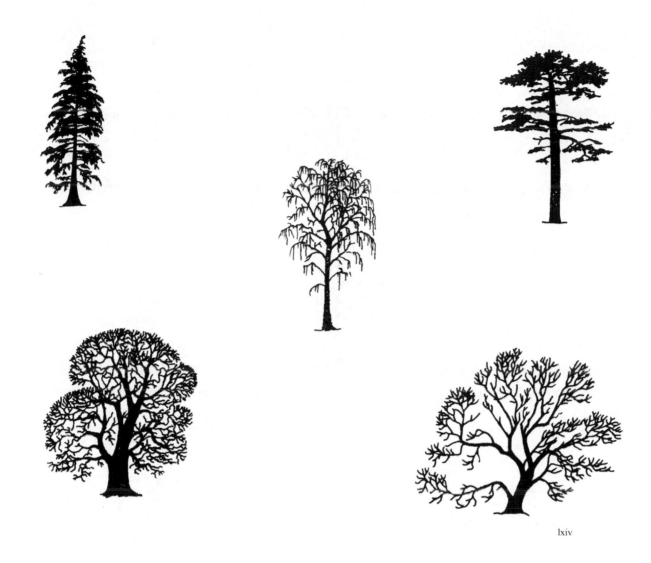

1. Draw a line on the right side of all the trees with needles.

2. Draw a star on the top of the pine tree that looks the most like a Christmas tree.

3. Put a check below the three trees that have no leaves or needles.

4. Draw an X through the trees on the bottom and circle the tree in the middle.

5. Draw a line from the tree in the middle to both trees on the top of the page.

Multiple Step Directions with Images

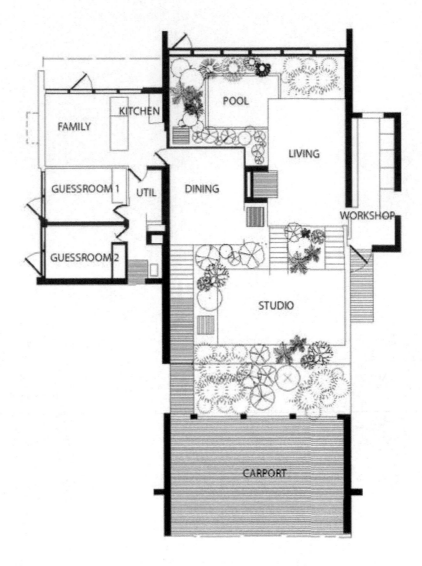

1. Draw a car in the carport facing down.

2. Write the letter B in the living room and the letter Q in the pool.

3. Draw a line from the kitchen, through the dining room and into the workshop.

4. Put and X in all the rooms that start with a letter that comes before O in the alphabet.

5. Draw two Xs to the left of the house and an O to the right of the house.

Multiple Step Directions with Images

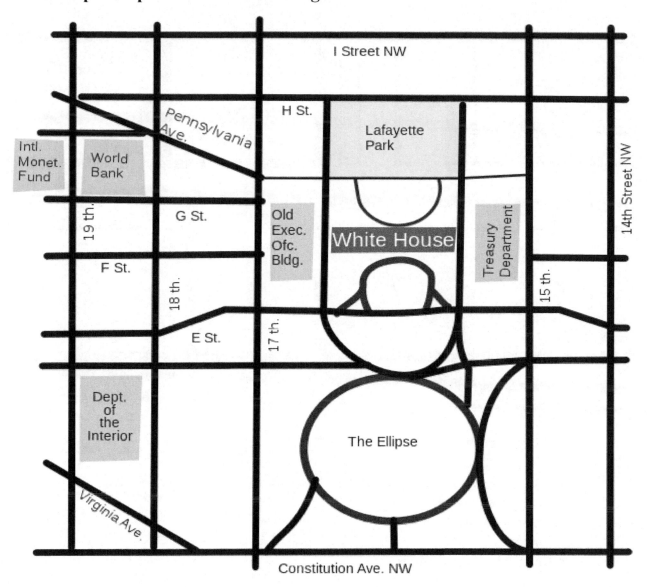

1. Draw a star at the intersection of 18th Street and E Street.

2. Make a zigzag line from the World Bank to the Department of the Interior following 19th street.

3. Put on X at the intersection of 15th street and H street. From the X, draw a line diagonally through Lafayette Park to the Old Executive Office Building.

Multiple Step Directions with Images

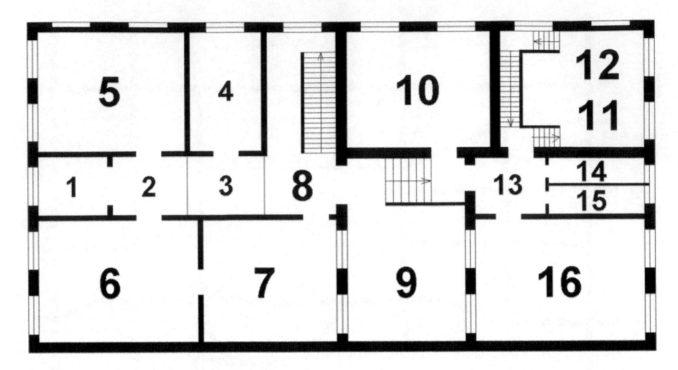

1. Circle all the even numbers.

2. Draw a line connecting all the numbers divisible by three starting with 15.

3. Put an X on all the staircases.

4. Draw a bed in 3 of the large rooms.

5. Make a path from room #5 to room #16.

6. Write the letter I in all the inner rooms.

7. Underline all the odd numbers.

8. Put a star in the doorways of all corner rooms.

9. Make a path connecting room #14 with room #1.

10. Add a zero at the end of all the double digit numbers and put a 1 before all the single

    digit numbers.

Comprehension of Factual Sentences: Yes/No

1. An average male spends around 3,100 hours of his life shaving.

   -Does an average male spend around 3,100 hours of his life showering?

2. The average person eats 4 spiders every year in their sleep.

   -Does the average person eat 12 spiders in their sleep a year?

3. Most people shed between 50 to 100 hairs every day.

   -Do most people shed over 50 hairs every day?

4. Jupiter is the largest planet in our solar system.

   - Is Mars the largest planet in our solar system?

5. Squirrels forget where they've hidden 50% of their nuts.

   Do Squirrels remember where they hide 50% of their nuts?

6. The first bullet proof vest was invented by a woman.

   -Did a man invent the first bullet proof vest?

7. Cold weather makes fingernails grow faster.

   -Do fingernails grow faster in cold weather?

8. Mohammad is the most common name in the world.

   -Is John the most common name in the world?

9. It takes about 7 minutes for the average person to fall asleep.

   -Is it about average to fall asleep in 17 minutes?

10. You can give change for a dollar in 293 coin variations.

   -Are there 239 ways you can give change for a dollar?

Comprehension of Factual Sentences: Yes/No

1. It takes 13 hours to build a Toyota and 6 months to build a Rolls Royce.

   Does it take longer to build a Toyota than a Rolls Royce?

2. A cat's ear has a total of thirty two muscles.

   Does a cat's ear have more than twenty five muscles?

3. The average person laughs 15 times a day.

   Is it above average to laugh 7 times a day?

4. The eye of an ostrich is larger than it's brain.

   Does an ostrich have a big brain?

5. Ants can lift 50 times their own weight.

   Is an ant strong?

6. It is impossible to fold a piece of paper in half more than 7 times.

   Can you fold a piece of paper in half 6 times?

7. More people are killed from donkeys in a year than in plane accidents.

   Are donkeys deadlier than airplanes?

8. Dust in your house consists mostly of dead skin.

   Does household dust consist mostly of dirt?

9. The first owner of the cigarette company Marlboro died of lung cancer.

   Did Marlboro's first owner die in a car crash?

10. It takes a fully loaded supertanker 20 minutes to come to a complete stop.

    Can supertankers stop quickly?

Comprehension of Factual Sentences: Yes/No

1. One fifth of all publications from Japan are comic books.

   -Are over half of the publications from Japan comic books?

2. Four out of five people over 100 years old are women.

   -Are 80% of people over 100 years old women?

3. The Titanic ship cost 7 million dollars to make, while the movie *Titanic* cost 200 million dollars to produce.

   -Did the ship cost more to make than the move?

4. Mercury is the only metal that is liquid when it is at room temperature.

   -Is Mercury a liquid at room temperature?

5. The only animal with four knees is an elephant.

   -Does an rhinoceros have four knees?

6. Snails can sleep for up to 3 years.

   - Can snails live longer than two years?

7. The Sears Tower in Chicago has enough steel to build 50,000 automobiles.

   -Are automobiles constructed of steel?

8. The steepest street in the world, Baldwin Street, is located in Dunedin, New Zealand.

   - Is San Francisco's Filbert Street the steepest street in the world?

9. The only flying saucer launch pad is located in Alberta Canada.

   - Is there such a thing as a flying saucer launch pad?

10. Only humans cry because of feelings.

    - Do cats cry when they are sad?

Comprehension of Factual Sentences: Yes/No

1. YKK is the worlds largest zipper manufacturer and makes 7.2 billion zippers a year.

- Does your zipper have YKK on it?

2. There are more chickens than humans in the world.

- Are chickens an endangered species?

3. The hottest continent on earth is Africa, with a record high of 136.4 degrees F.

-Is the hottest continent on earth Africa?

4. Mount Everest is the tallest mountain in the world at 29,028 feet high.

-Is Mount Everest taller than Mt. McKinley?

5. The heaviest baby born weighed 22 lb 8 oz and was born in Italy in September 1955.

-Did the heaviest baby weigh more than 22 lbs?

6. About 20 percent of the Earth's land is made up of desert.

- Is the majority of the Earth desert?

7. Lake Baikal in Russia is the deepest lake in the world and holds as much water as all the five Great Lakes of the U.S. combined!

- Does Lake Erie have more water than Lake Baikal?

8. Jupiter is a planet made entirely of gases.

- Does Jupiter consist of only gases?

9. The Empire State Building once got stuck by lightning 9 times in 20 minutes.

- Did the Empire State Building get struck by lightning more than 6 times?

10. The only food that doesn't spoil is honey.

- Does honey go bad after 6 months?

Comprehension of Factual Sentences: Yes/No

1. Thomas Edison, the inventor of the light bulb, was afraid of the dark.

-Did Thomas Edison like the dark?

2. It is impossible to sneeze with your eyes open.

- Can you sneeze with your eyes closed?

3. Babe Ruth kept a cabbage leaf under his cap to keep cool.

-Did Babe Ruth keep a lettuce leaf under his cap?

4. Vincent Van Gogh only sold one painting while he was alive.

- Did only one person ever purchase Van Gogh's art?

5. Water is the only substance on earth that is lighter as a solid than as a liquid.

- Is ice heavier than the same amount of water?

6. When an octopus gets angry, it shoots a stream of black ink.

- Does an octopus shoot ink when it is angry?

7. The lung fish can live out of water for as long as four years.

-Does the lung fish require water at all times to survive ?

8. The only bird that can fly backwards is the hummingbird.

- Can a dove fly backwards?

9. Tigers have striped skin, not just striped fur.

- Do Tigers have striped skin?

10. A skunk can spray its stench twelve feet away.

- Are you safe from a skunk's spray if you stand 10 feet away?

Comprehension of Factual Sentences: Yes/No

1. In one day, your heart beats 100,000 times.

- Does your heart beat 100,000 times in an hour?

2. Half your body's red blood cells are replaced every seven days.

- Do half of the red blood cells in your body get replaced every week?

3. A human's blood vessels stretched out could go around the world twice.

- If you stretched out all of your blood vessels, could they go around the world twice?

4. 85% of the population can curl their tongue into a tube.

- Can the majority of the population curl their tongue?

5. Pinocchio means "pine head" in Italian.

- Does the word Pinocchio mean "pine head" in Spanish?

6. Anatidaephobia is the fear that, somewhere out there, a duck is watching you.

- Is Anatidaephobia the fear that a duck is watching you?

7. Honey bees have hair on their eyes.

- Do honey bees have hair on their eyes?

8. The mayfly only lives for 8 hours.

- Can a mayfly see the sunrise and set?

9. The more salt you put on ice, the more the ice melts.

- Does salt make ice melt?

10. A lightning bolt is 4 times hotter than the sun.

- Is the sun hotter than lightning?

Comprehension of Factual Sentences: Yes/No

1. Africa is the continent with the most countries.

   -Does Asia have more countries than Africa?

2. Bacteria are the most common organism on earth.

   - Are there more bacteria than humans?

3. Alaska is the U.S. State with the largest coastline.

   -Does California have a larger coast than Alaska?

4. In 1887, a snowflake in Montana was 15 inches wide.

   - Was the snowflake wider than a foot?

5. Chandra Bahadur Dangi of Nepal is the world's shortest man, 21.5 inches tall.

   -Is he over 2 feet tall?

6. The first animal sent to outer space was a dog.

   -Was a dog the first animal sent to space?

7. It takes Mercury only 88 days to circle the sun, the length of a year on Mercury.

   -Does the Earth circle the sun faster than Mercury?

8. Cats are North America's most popular pets: there are 73 million cats compared to 63 million dogs. Over 30% of the households in North America have a cat.

   -Do the majority of households in North American have cats?

9. Humans can survive longer without food than they can without sleep.

   - Is sleep more essential to humans for survival than food?

10. It takes a glass bottle over 500 years to biodegrade.

    - If you throw away a glass bottle, will it still be in the ground when you die?

Comprehension of Detailed Factual Sentences

1. Everyone has a unique tongue print in addition to their finger print to identify them.

   - What print can be used to identify a person instead of a finger print?

2. Humans shed about 1.5 lbs of skin every year. By the time someone reaches age 70, they will have lost over 100 lbs of skin.

   - What do human shed over 100 lbs of in their lifetime?

3. Babies are born with 350 bones. As we age, bones fuse together and adults grow to have only 206 bones.

   - Whose bodies contain 350 bones?

4. The small intestine is between 18-24 feet long.

   - What human organ is longer than 17 feet?

5. Dogs circle the floor before they lie down because they are hardwired to exhibit this behavior. Their ancestors circled in the woods or grass to make a soft bed to lie in.

   - Why do dogs circle the floor before they lie down?

6. A human sneeze can expel air at speeds of up to 100 miles per hour.

   - How fast can the air from a human sneeze travel?

7. The average person creates enough saliva to fill two swimming pools in their lifetime.

    - What does the average person create enough of to fill two swimming pools?

8. The great white shark rolls its eyes into the back of its head when it attacks prey in order

    to protect its eyes from thrashing and the inevitable debris.

    - What does the great white shark do with its eyes when it attacks?

9. Americans consumed 76 billion pounds of red meat and poultry in the year 2000, up

    21% from a decade earlier.

    - When did Americans consume 76 billion pounds of red meat and poultry?

10. The Kiwi, the national bird of New Zealand, lives in the ground, lays only one egg a

    year, is nearly blind and can't fly. It has survived for 70 million years.

    - What country does the Kiwi bird live in?

11. There are more public libraries in the U.S. than McDonald's, a total of 15,946 libraries

    compared to 14,000 McDonald's.

    - How many public libraries are there in there in the U.S.?

12. An electric Japanese toilet seat newly available in the U.S. for $800 offers deluxe

    comforts including: heating, a water spray, fan and antibacterial glazing.

    - How much does the luxury toilet seat cost?

Comprehension of Detailed Factual Information

1. The Great Pyramid of Egypt, built about 2600 BC, was constructed with enough stone to make a brick wall 20 inches high that could go around the world.

   - When was the Great Pyramid of Egypt Built?

   - What material is the Great Pyramid made of?

2. Alabama is the only state with all major natural resources needed to make iron and steel. It is also the largest supplier of cast-iron and steel pipe products.

   - What does Alabama have the natural resources to make?

   - What is Alabama the largest supplier of?

3. Eating asparagus will make your urine have a pungent odor as soon as 15 minutes after consumption. During digestion, the vegetable's sulfurous amino acids break down into odorous chemical components which not everybody can smell but are present in all urine after asparagus consumption.

   - How soon after eating asparagus will urine have a pungent odor?

   - Is everybody able to smell the odor?

4. Ocean tides are caused by the combined effects of the gravitational forces exerted by the moon and sun, as well as the rotation of the earth, to make the sea level rise and fall.

   -What two things cause tides?

   - What is an ocean tide?

Comprehension of Details: Advertisements

1. Two lost puppies: 11 week old female boxer spayed and micro-chipped and male boxer neutered and micro-chipped. Last seen near Elm Park. $500 reward for safe return.

   - What breed of dog is missing?

   -Where were they last seen?

   - How much is the reward for finding them?

   - Do the dogs have identification?

2. For Sale: 1990 Chevrolet Corvette 6 speed manual. In excellent condition with 48,000 original miles. Asking $9,999.

   -What year is the automobile?

   -What make?

   - How many miles are on it?

   - How much does it cost?

3. Garage Sale: Saturday April 12th from 7am until 12pm. Selling: exercise equipment, baby boy clothes, toys, books, movies, household items and much more. Address: 600 Honeysuckle Lane, rain or shine.

   - What day is the garage sale?

   - When does it end?

   -Name three types of items for sale

   - Will they cancel the garage sale if it rains?

Comprehension of Details: Advertisements

4. Clothing Drive: In desperate need of winter clothing for women and children. Accepting clothing for newborn to teenagers for both boys and girls. Also need crib bedding and infant feeding accessories. Drop off between 5-7 at St. Stephen's Church, 502 Elm Rd. January 5th through the 8th.

   - What items do they need?

   - Where should you drop them off?

   - What time can you drop the items off?

   - What are the days of the clothing drive?

5. Guitar Lessons: Beginners welcome. I have guitars you can learn on. Learn chords, structure, scales, music reading and song writing. I have 18 years of experience in blues, folk and rock. Lessons are $25 an hour. Available evening, weekends and Thursday afternoons. Call Tom: (703) 522 3489.

   - Do you need to bring your own guitar?

   - How much are lessons?

   - Does Tom have experience with classical music?

   - Is he available for lessons on Thursday afternoons?

   - What is Tom's area code?

Comprehension of Details: Advertisements

6. Beautiful pug puppies are ready for a new home. 8 weeks old. $300 each. They both have all of their shots. Call Mary after 5pm. (821) 348 5911

   - What breed of dog is for sale?

   - How old are they?

   - Do they have all their shots?

   -Can you call Mary about the pugs in the morning?

7. Personals: I am looking for a female that lives or works in the downtown Chicago area that would like to get together for lunch or dinner sometime. Looking for somewhat of a regular thing where we get together for meals, have some conversation and get to know each other. I am a 35 year old white male, corporate type (clean-cut), with no drama or nonsense. I look for you to be decent, with a good head on your shoulders between 25 and 40 years old. Race is not an issue. If you want to know more, respond so we can get to know each other.

   - Where does he live?

   - Is he interested in women under 25?

   - How old is he?

   - Does he like to wear ripped jeans, hats and sloppy clothing?

Comprehension of Details: Advertisements

8. Personals: Hello, I'm a mother of two beautiful kids in the Richmond, VA area. I'm looking for a laid back male who knows how to treat a women and will accept my kids. You have to be good looking, have a good job and have your things together. I'm huge on romance so please be romantic. I love a man that can cook. If you meet what I'm asking for, please respond with a photo and I'll send one back :).

- Where does she live?

- How many children does she have?

- Can her potential date be unemployed?

- Would she be interested in a first date if he offers to cook for her?

- Does her date need to like kids?

9. Roommate Wanted: Park Ridge subdivision. $500 a month. Upstairs furnished room with large bedroom, sitting area, and bathroom. Home is conveniently located near the hospital and the mall. Cable, wireless internet, washer and dryer and all utilities are included. Looking for Male or Female who is responsible, clean, and working. Home is smoke free, well maintained and quiet.

- Is it a house or apartment?

- Are cable and internet included?

- How much is the rent?

-Will you need to furnish the room?

- Will they rent to a male roommate?

Comprehension of Details: Advertisements

10. Vacation Rental: 2 bedroom, 2 Bath Myrtle Beach vacation rental. Two blocks from the beach. Golf cart, washer & dryer, gas grill and hot tub included. January through May, weekly rate: $600.00, daily rate: $86.00 June through September, weekly rate:$1200, week of July 4th: $1400.

- What comes with the vacation rental?

-Where is it located?

- How much will it cost to rent it for a week in April?

-How much will it cost to rent the week of July 4th?

11. Immaculate home available for rent: 3,100 square feet for $2,500 a month. Incredible upgrades throughout entire home. Features 2 story foyer, 4 bedrooms, 3 full baths, bonus room, 2 car garage with door opener, dining room, family room with gas fireplace, office, and living room. The gourmet kitchen has a wall oven, stainless steel appliances, and island. There are wood floors throughout and home stereo system. Fenced backyard with two locking gates and lots of privacy with nature preserve to side and back of house.

- How many square feet is the home?

- What is the monthly rent?

- Does it have a fenced backyard?

- How many bedrooms is it?

- What type of kitchen appliances does it have?

Comprehension of Details: Advertisements

12. For Sale: 2001 Harley Davidson Fatboy (Fuel injected). My wife says it has to go. It has just under 32k miles. Stays in the garage and kept clean. Lots of chrome. Paint scheme is black and yellow. Priced $1000 below value at $8250, looking to sell quickly. Never been laid down or wrecked. Tires are in great shape and has a new battery. Rides great!

-Why is he selling his Harley Davidson?

- What year is it?

- What is the asking price?

- Has it been in an accident?

- How many miles are on it?

- According to the owner, what is the actual value of the motorcycle?

13. For Sale: Old antique two person saw: Asking $250 or best offer . Also have a small antique saw for $50, antique metal signs for $20 each and some old antique wash boards. All of the items are in great condition. If interested, please call or text George at 880-829-9521. I will send pictures on request.

-What is for sale?

-How much is the two person saw?

- Will he accept $225 if it is the best offer?

- How much does he want for each antique metal signs?

- Who is selling them?

- What is the phone number?

Comprehension of Details: Advertisements

14. For Sale: Thomas the Train set for $450. I have combined 5 Thomas sets, additional tracks plus accessories to create this set. Set will include all of the extra tracks and accessories, over 15 trains, scenery mat, stop light, clock tower with bridge, Cranky the Crane and lots of extra trees. Also, motorized Thomas the Train and the motorized jet. Table is not included but negotiable. In excellent condition. All items are functioning. I would give it a 9.5 out of 10 in condition. I spent over $1200 for the set.

- How much is the set?

- Is the train table included?

- Does the set include over 20 trains?

- How much did the set cost retail?

15. For Sale: Novus Zero Gravity Recliner, $1800. I bought it at the Relax the Back store in St. Louis. It is dark brown leather and has power recline, power retractable footrest and adjustable lumbar support. Purchase price was $3104. It still has a four year factory warranty. I bought this chair for my teenage son who had back surgery. He used it for a week, got better and has not used it since. It is in absolutely perfect condition. This is a great chair for anyone and clearly it is the very best for anyone with back pain.

- How much is the recliner?

- What did they pay for it brand new?

- How long did her son use it?

Comprehension of Details: Advertisements

16. For Sale: Cow Skull $45. This hand painted ceramic cow skull has a rustic, crackled finish, very old and worn look. Approximately, 20" x 20" x 9" deep. rabbit fur, concho and beads complete the look. It would make a great Christmas gift for someone who loves rustic, western, Native American decor. call 734-254-0221 no texting please.

- What is for sale?

- How many inches deep is it?

- What is the skull decorated with?

17. For Sale: Riding mower with a 17.5 Briggs and Stratton motor and a 42" cutting deck. This mower just received a complete tune up with a new air filter, new spark plug, oil change, blades were sharpened and balanced. The mower also had a brand new cutting belt installed and the battery is less than a year old. Runs like new and cuts evenly . I have done everything to insure you can go pick up leaves and cut grass trouble free. This mower was used on a quarter acre for only two seasons. $625.00. NO EMAILS OR TEXTS PHONE CALLS ONLY. 981-216-1992 NO CALLS AFTER 9 PM PLEASE!!!!

- What was done to tune up the mower?

- How much does it cost?

- Can you text him for information?

-How late can you call to ask about the mower?

-How old is the battery?

Comprehension of Details: Advertisements

18. Babysitter: I am looking to babysit in my home east of Atlanta. I have several years of childcare experience, both in professional centers as well as in my home. I would offer one-on-one time with your child, reading, crafts and playing outside. I would also be able to provide nutritious food for your child. I've worked in elementary school cafeterias and took several child nutrition courses. My rate is $85 a day, including meals & snacks. If you are looking for a safe, fun and educational place for your child, please contact me.

- Is the sitter offering to babysit outside her own home?

- How much does it cost a day?

- Are meals and snacks extra?

- Name three things the babysitter will do with your child.

19. For Sale: Large Kobalt tool box and tools. 36" wide, 18" deep, 64" high. Has built-in power strip, heavy duty locking wheels, coat hooks, separate locking key/wallet drawer. Like new condition. Box is filled with Snap-on and Craftsman tools. Includes: air gun, air ratchet, air chisel, air grinder, air drill, sockets ¼ " and ½" sockets and adapters. Wrenches include both metric and standard sets. Many other miscellaneous tools, $2,000.00 firm or trade for good-running, gas-efficient automobile

- Is the tool box taller than 3 feet?

- Name three types of tools included.

- What will the seller accept as a trade for the toolbox?

Comprehension of Details: Advertisements

20. Nana's Pet Sitting is looking for pet sitters and dog walkers in Manhattan. Background check must be squeaky clean. Must have a cell phone, computer with internet access, printer and reliable transportation. This is a fun job for a person who loves animals and the outdoors. You will also learn excellent pet care skills, pet first aid and CPR. We have a great team of awesome pet sitters and dog walkers! If you would like to join us and you offer honesty, integrity and reliability, then please contact us right away. Pay is $10 per dog for half hour walk, $25 dollars a day for pet sitting in your own home.

-What is the job?

-Where is the job located?

- Name five things required for the job.

- Will they do a background check?

- What skill will the pet sitting company teach you?

- If you walk 3 dogs at a time and do a total of 5 half hour walks a day, how much will you make?[1]

- If you watch two dogs in your home for 10 days, how much will you earn?[2]

---

1   $150
2   $500

Comprehension of Details: Advertisements

21. Wellness Chef Position:

The Center for Meditation and Well-Being is searching for a chef to prepare meals for wellness and meditation retreats, retreat center guests and staff.

Responsibilities include: preparing menus and meals for guests and staff, ordering and maintaining kitchen inventory, overseeing cleanliness and health standards, coordinating volunteers and staff, and cultivating a harmonious work environment. The retreat center is nestled on a mountain peak of stunning natural beauty in the Smokey Mountains. The spiritual center and spa cherishes family, service and silence. Benefits include: retreats at discounted rates, participation in yoga and meditation sessions, and retreat center accommodations. Financial package to be commensurate with skills and experience. The ideal candidate will possess skills in vegetarian cooking, preferably in raw, Indian and/or Ayurvedic food prep, several years prior cooking experience, and experience cooking for groups from 20-100 people. Resumes can be emailed. Our office can be reached from 9:30am-5:30pm Wednesday through Monday.

- Where is the meditation retreat located?

- What type of food will the cook be expected to prepare?

- What size group should the cook have experience cooking for?

- In addition to cooking, what are some of the job responsibilities?

-What three things does the spiritual center cherish?

- What benefits come with the job?

- Can you call the office on Tuesday at 10 am?

Comprehension of Details: Advertisements

22. PROGRAM SPECIALIST / LIVE ANIMAL MANAGER

Position available at the Museum of Natural History for informal educator needed to develop and present natural science programs for students and general audiences. Typical activities include: making educational presentations, program development and the facilitation of public events, workshops and special classes. The Program Specialist will also manage the museum's live animal collection in support of exhibits and programs. This responsibility includes: daily care and feeding of animals, purchasing supplies, maintaining health records and permits. Position also requires the maintenance and supervision of live animal staff and volunteers. This position requires a four-year degree from an accredited university in education, zoology, natural science, biology or a related field. Experience with live animals including mammals, reptiles, fish and invertebrates is required. Museum or interpretative facility education experience is preferred. Candidate must possess a valid driver's license and good driving record. Public presentation skills are essential. Position requires a flexible work schedule that will include some evenings, weekends and holidays. Teacher certification is preferred but not required. Drug screening required. Salary: $30,000 - $36,000, depending on experience. Interested applicants should email a resume and letter of interest, no calls or drop-ins will be considered.

Program specialist/ Live Animal Manager, Museum of Natural History:

Questions:

1. What degree is required for this position?

2. To be considered for this job, what should you have studied in college?

3. What are the responsibilities of the job?

4. Will you supervise staff and volunteers?

5. Must you have a teachers certification?

6. What is the salary range?

7. Will you be required to work some evenings, weekends and holidays?

8. If you are afraid of snakes, is this job a good fit?

9. Is experience with live animals including fish, reptiles, mammals and invertebrates preferred or required?

10. Will a fear of public speaking impact your performance on the job?

11. Will they conduct a drug screening?

12. Is driving part of the job requirements?

13. Can you apply by calling?

14. What museum has the job opening?

15. Is it a good idea to drop in to be considered for the job?

Comprehension of Details: Advertisements

23. Schwinn legacy cruiser bike for sale, $100. It is intended for women aged 17 years and up. Its sleek design and curved lines give this light blue and white bike a classic look. This slim bike is sturdy and durable. It is a 1-speed bike and has a rear coaster brake system for quick and safe stops. The bike has a steel bicycle chain, front fender, spokes and plastic pedals. This woman's cruiser bike has 26" front and rear wheels with metal alloy rims. The included kickstand allows for easy parking. The seat has a spring construction and cushioned top to offer firm support and comfort. It has a maximum weight capacity of 300 lbs. I have owned this bike for about six months and LOVE it. I'm only selling because I'm preparing to move out of state and it's not cost-effective to bring the bike. I also have a matching men's Schwinn cruiser available and would entertain a discount for buying them together.

- What brand is the bike?

- How much is it?

- How big are the wheels?

- Can somebody who is 325 lbs ride it?

- How many speeds is the bike?

- Does it have a kick stand?

- What color is it?

- Why is she selling it?

-What else does she have to sell?

Comprehension of Details: Advertisements

24. Male vocalist wanted. We are a very busy established wedding/corporate/festival band with lots of bookings well into the next year and a half. Looking for a experienced singer for Soul, Motown, Beach, 70's, 80s to current variety band. We are seeking a good vocalist and someone who can move well and dance in order to put on a good visual show. Great pay up to $400 a gig. We provided transportation and are looking for someone who is easy to work with and has experience with performing. We provide all the band equipment. We wear matching tuxedos when we perform but we will cover half the cost of your tuxedo.

- Do they need a male or female singer?

- Do you need to have experience?

- Is it okay if you can't dance?

- How much do you get paid for each show?

- What type of music will you be singing?

- What sorts of events does the band perform for?

- Will you need any equipment?

- Will you need to pay the whole cost for your tuxedo?

Comprehension of Details: Advertisements

25. Make Up Artist: I am a Freelance/Mobile Makeup Artist. I provide makeup services for makeovers, weddings, photo shoots, fashion shows, birthday parties and special effects.

My rate are as follows:

Travel Expense: $20	Makeovers: $25
Eyelashes: $10	Eyebrow Contouring: $10
Bridal: $65 Bride	$50 for each Bridesmaid

- How much are makeovers for a wedding with 4 bridesmaids and travel expenses?[3]

- How much will makeovers cost for a bachelorette party of 12? [4]

- What company does she work for?

26. Larry's Landscaping and Lawn Care Inc. will be out delivering fresh cut Fraser fir Christmas trees to your door. We are offering 6 to 9 ft trees delivered to your door from $35 and up. We bring a selection of trees for you to choose from. Stands are $15 and set up in your home is an additional $10.

- How tall are the Christmas trees?

- What type of trees are they?

- Where do you go to purchase the trees?

- How much extra is a tree stand?

- What is the total cost for their lowest price tree, a stand and set up?[5]

---

3 $285
4 $300
5 $60

Comprehension of Factual Paragraphs: Who, What and When.

1. Marie Curie discovered the elements polonium and radium. She was awarded two Nobel Prizes. She died in On July 4, 1934 from radiation poisoning as a result of her extensive work with X-Rays.

- Who discovered polonium?

- What other element did she discover?

- When did she die?

2. Before the 1860s, people did not understand what caused disease. Louis Pasteur, a french chemist, experimented with bacteria and discovered that disease came from microorganisms. He also found that bacteria could be killed with disinfectant and exposure to high temperatures. After his discovery, doctors began to wash their hands and sterilize their instruments preventing infection and the spread of disease.

- Who discovered diseases came from microorganisms?

- What did he discover could killed bacteria?

- When did Louis Pasteur make his discoveries?

Comprehension of Factual Paragraphs: Who, What and When.

1. In 1922, Richard Gurley Drew, a 3M engineer, invented masking tape in St. Paul. Minnesota. By 1930, he perfected his waterproof, see through sticky tape, "Scotch" tape. It was immediately popular during the great depression, helping people repair items instead of having to purchase something new.

- Who invented scotch tape?

- What is scotch tape?

- When was scotch tape invented?

2. Morphine was first discovered and used as a pain killer in 1804 by the chemist Friedrich Serturner. He was the first person able to isolate an alkaloid from a plant. He began distributing morphine as a pain killer in 1817 and in 1827 Merick sold it commercially. Merick was a small chemist shop at that time. Serturner originally named the drug Morphium after the Greek God of dreams, Morpheus, because of the its tendency to cause sleep.[lxviii]

-Who discovered Morphine?

- When was it invented?

- What is it used for?

- Who was it named after?

Comprehension of Paragraphs

Chocolate Chip Cookies

Chocolate chip cookies are a favorite treat around the world but have only been in existence since the 1930s. They were invented by Ruth Wakerfield. She was born in 1905 and grew up to be a dietician and food lecturer. She and her husband Kenneth bought a tourist lodge named the Toll House Inn, where she prepared recipes for meals that were served to guests.

In 1930, Wakefield was mixing a batch of cookies for her guests when she discovered that she was out of baker's chocolate. She substituted broken pieces of Nestle's semi-sweet chocolate, expecting it to melt and absorb into the dough to create chocolate cookies. That didn't happen. When she removed the pan from the oven, Wakefield realized that she had accidentally invented "chocolate chip cookies". Her guest loved them and they became a staple at the inn.

She called them "Toll House Crunch Cookies". They became extremely popular locally and the recipe was soon published in a Boston newspaper. They became a favorite component of care packages sent to soldiers in World War II. The sales of Nestle chocolates increases as chocolate chip cookies became more and more popular. Nestle's Chocolates worked out an agreement with Ruth Wakefield. Nestle would print the Toll House Cookie recipe on its package, and Wakefield would be given a lifetime supply of Nestle chocolate. Thanks to her baking ingenuity, the chocolate chip cookie has become the most popular variety of cookie in America.[lxix]

Chocolate Chip Cookie: Questions

1. Who invented chocolate chip cookies?

2. When did she invent them?

3. What was her payment from Nestle for the invention?

4. Where did the name Nestle Toll House Chocolate Chip Cookies come from?

5. What was Ruth Wakefield's educational training?

6. What city's newspaper was her recipe published in?

7. Did Ruth Wakerfield set out to make chocolate chip cookies?

8. During what war did soldiers enjoy receiving chocolate chip cookies in their care packages?

Comprehension of News Articles

Two women are out of the hospital after a collision with a moose Friday. But there's a very unusual twist: one of the women was jogging when the moose hit her. An Anchorage County's Sheriff's Department spokesman says the accident happened around 6 pm on southbound Pleasant Parkway near the ramp to the Elm Greenway. A 81-year-old woman was driving an SUV when the moose stepped into the roadway and hit the front passenger side of her car. The impact sent the moose airborne and it hit a 19-year-old female jogger who was running on a path. Both women were taken to the hospital for treatment and released from the hospital Monday. Unfortunately, the moose didn't survive the accident.

- How many cars were involved in the accident?

- Were there any casualties?

- What happened to the jogger?

- How old was the driver?

- How old was the jogger?

- How many days were the women in the hospital?

Comprehension of News Articles

A Italian Airlines flight suffered a technical malfunction and made an emergency landing in Paris, injuring 49 people. Five people were seriously hurt and one critically injured. A problem with the right engine of the Boeing 747 forced the plane to make an emergency landing. It was a rough landing and the right side of the plane hit the tarmac at the International Airport in Paris. The authorities said 28 of the injured people were treated at the airport while 21 others were transported to the hospital. A spokesman for the airlines said five people were seriously injured amid the mad scramble to evacuate the plane. The flight, arriving from Rome before dawn, was transporting 315 passengers and originally was destined for London.

- Where was the flight coming from?

- Where did it have to make an emergency landing?

- What was wrong with the plane?

- What type of plane was it?

- Was anybody critically injured?

- How were some passengers injured?

- Where were the passengers hoping to land?

- How many people were injured?

- Was everybody on the plane hurt?

Comprehension of News Articles

An Atlantic City taxi driver returned $400,000 left in his cab by a big-time poker player. He was rewarded for the good deed with $20,000 cash. Al Savino, the cab driver, had more than 14 years of experience on the job in Atlantic City.

The poker player had left behind a black leather suitcase stuffed with cash when Savino dropped him off at the Harrah's Resort and Spa. The doorman at Savino's next stop alerted him to the bag, and when the taxi driver opened it, he pulled out about $50,000 in cash. He put back the money and called dispatch right away to get the name of his previous passenger and alert them to the situation. He returned to his previous stop at Harrah's Resort and was able to locate the grateful owner of the suitcase.

The next day the poker player called the taxi company and gave Al Savino $20,000 for returning the suitcase that contained over $400,000 in cash.

The taxi company also rewarded Savino with the title Driver of the Year, $1,000 and a dinner for two at a five star restaurant.

- How much money was in the suitcase?

- What is the name of the taxi driver?

- How did the driver find the name of the poker player who left the suitcase in his car?

- How much did the owner of the suitcase give Al?

- Where was the poker player dropped off?

- What did the taxi company do?

- In total, how much was Al rewarded for his honest deed?

Comprehension of News Articles

A "polar vortex", a whirlpool of frigid air, descended Sunday onto much of the U.S., pummeling parts of the country with a dangerous cold that could break records that are decades old with wind chill warnings stretching from Montana to Florida.

For a large portion of the Midwest, the subzero temperatures were moving in behind another winter storm front that carried more than a foot of snow and high winds that made traveling extremely dangerous. Officials closed schools in cities including Chicago, St. Louis, Cleveland and Milwaukee and warned residents to stay indoors and avoid the frigid cold altogether.

The forecast is extreme and predicts 32 below zero temperatures in Fargo, North Dakota, 21 below zero in Madison, Wisconsin and 15 below zero in Minneapolis, Indianapolis and Chicago. Wind chills factor into what the temperature feels like with the addition of the cold wind, and could drop into the minus 50s and 60s.

   - What is the extreme weather system called?

   - Name three cities where there are already school closings.

   - What is the predicted temperature for Fargo, North Dakota?

   - Should people spend time outdoors?

   - What is the predicted wind chill temperature?

   - How much snow accumulated in the earlier winter storm?

Comprehension of News Articles

A 77-year-old great-grandfather in Montgomery County has been charged in connection with a murder-for-hire case. Albert Smith of the 500 block of Oak Road was charged Tuesday with solicitation to commit murder, officials said.

Smith allegedly offered Ted Walton $3,500 to shoot an acquaintance who owed him $10,000, reported the chief deputy in the Montgomery County sheriff's office.

Walton reported the incident to authorities on Monday, and Smith was arrested the next day. They acted quickly to prevent someone from being hurt or killed. Smith was placed in the county jail on $750,000 bond and has his first court appearance on Monday.

His wife, Sarah, said Thursday that she is trying to understand the charges against her husband. She said the charges are out of character for the man shes been married to for 54 years. "I am absolutely shocked," gasped Sarah Smith. She said her husband is a retired electrician who has had back, heart and other health problems. He also has had recent memory problems.

- Does Albert Smith have any children?

- How much money did his acquaintance owe him?

- How much did Smith offer Walton for the shooting?

- Did Walton shoot the man for Smith?

- How much is Smith's bond?

- How long have Sarah and Albert been married?

Comprehension of Short Stories

Excerpt from *Running Wire at the Front Lines* by Louis Lauria

Dud

On this one particular day, we were in position in a field about two hundred yards wide with trees outlining it on all sides. The cannons were spaced out as always about ten to fifteen yards apart. For awhile, there was a lull in the fighting. Some of the boys got into their foxholes and tried to get some needed sleep which was hard to get. Some men would just mope around and others would pick up a *Stars and Stripes* newspaper and read.

After about one hour, some mortar and artillery shells came in on us. Steve and I were up at the observation post and got word that the guns were getting attacked. The shells exploded in the gun section within ten and twenty yards apart. Up at the O.P., we looked to see where the enemy guns were firing from. Another barrage of shells came in. They were exploding close but we couldn't seem to locate the guns. About 15 more rounds came in after this. All of a sudden, one of the men in the gun section started to scream. It was sharp and shrill and he repeated it for some time. This made most of the cannon crew look out of their foxholes to see what was going on. This GI kept on screaming for a few more minutes. He tried to explain what happened and pointed to his foxhole but wouldn't go near it.

After he got his head together, he told everyone that a shell had landed between his legs while he was in a squat position. The shell had gone through his newspaper and his legs. The shell penetrated about a foot into the ground. As soon as this happened, he jumped out of the foxhole and started to scream.

Later, he realized how lucky he was to be alive. The shell was a dud. He thanked whoever made the shell. It must have been a prisoner of war. There were many of them helping in the war effort. They would do whatever they could to sabotage the enemy.

When I got back to the gun crew, I talked to the GI. He explained that when the shell hit he was so excited he jumped out of the foxhole in one leap as far as his legs would spring him, realizing the shell could be a time fuse. He thanked God for having a prisoner of war sabotage the shell. The Germans never could find out how many shells didn't explode. I guess this helped save a lot of our boys' lives. [lxx]

1. What landed in the trench?

2. Did it explode?

3. According to the author, why didn't the shell explode?

4. When do you think this took place?

5. What was the name of the newspaper that many of the GI read in the trenches?

6. Why was the GI screaming?

Comprehension of Short Stories

Excerpt from *Running Wire at the Front Lines* by Louis Lauria

Ring

My buddy Len gave me this German ring. He had gotten it off some other doughboy along the way. He came back to command post and had a few S, or what we called loot. I said, "Hey Len, how about giving me that ring you have." He stopped for a moment and said, "no." I asked again and again. Finally, he gave me the ring. He also had a German fountain pen. It was an old 14k gold pen with the old bladder which held the ink. I guess in those days it was worth something. Anyway, he gave me both of them.

After a few days, I asked him where he got the ring. I figured he looted it from inside a German house or had taken it from a German P.O.W. He said no it was given to him by one GI when he was up front at the OP. He then told me it came off a dead German's finger. I said, "What do you mean? He pulled it of his finger?" He said, "No, the GI had to cut it off the dead man's finger." After he told me that, I felt a little squeamish about the ring. After seeing so many dead Germans, I should have been used to this going on. I had gotten a cold sweat about the matter and wanted to give it back. Well, I didn't give it back. I put it inside the truck seat until the end of the war. I took it home with me but I always got that squeamish feeling about it. Sometimes, I would see it somewhere in my box of collections and say a prayer for whoever it belonged to. Sometimes I wanted to bury the ring. The ring is nice looking. It is gold and has an onyx stone.

I was never a GI who went looking in clothes of dead bodies for loot. I saw many other GIs search for loot in pockets of dead Krauts but I never had the guts for it. I saw more dead bodies than I want to talk about but never tried touching them. I have eaten within a few feet of them but never put my hand on them. I was always squeamish when it came to that sort of thing.[lxxi]

1.   Who gave him the ring?

2.   Where did it come from?

3.   What type of stone was in it?

4.   Did the author like the ring?

5.   What did he think of doing with the ring sometimes?

6.   What did the soldiers call loot?

7.   What else did Len give him?

Comprehension of Short Stories

Excerpt From *Running Wire at the Front Line* by Louis Lauria

Broken Teeth

On the second day of combat, I didn't know if the mortar or artillery shells were going or coming. My outfit was getting what was called battle of inoculation, which gave green troops a chance to get used to combat - something which I believe no one really ever get used to. We learned fast which shells belonged to the enemy and which ones were our own.

I was in my foxhole which was dug by the First Division men and decided to get out and walk around for a few minutes. I walked about ten feet away and was a bit afraid to go too far from my hole. Ten shells landed in the fields we occupied. I jumped up and leaped for my foxhole. I was so scared. I dove headfirst and hit my mouth on the side of the hole, which was about four feet deep. I was so frantic that I didn't realize that I hurt myself in the process. I didn't feel any pain after the incident since I was so scared. The impact loosened one of my front teeth.

After this accident, many months went by and there were never any signs of pain. I remember the weather had changed and it was starting to get cold. Winter approached. I bedded down for the night in a barn, and slept with a camel hair blanket. The night rang with gun fire . A GI woke me up in the middle of the night with the news to move forward to an observation post. I had such a bad pain on my front tooth. I tried to drink some coffee and eat some of my K-ration, but the pain was unbearable.

I asked my top Sergeant to go to the rear and see a dentist. He gave me the okay. A jeep driver drove me to the aid station. From there, I mounted a much larger truck with around ten

GIs who were also sick. We drove about forty miles or so away from the front lines. I guess that was the closest dentist around. When we did arrive, it had to be about three in the afternoon. I jumped off the truck and went into this building. It looked like a hospital. There were many GIs in clean olive drab. They were all doctors' aids. They stared at me with wide open eyes as if I walked in slow motion and in a real untidy appearance.

You must remember, I came from the front lines and not some fancy hotel. My shoes and pants were full of mud. My face looked just as bad. My face was swollen from pain and was very dirty. I may have never looked worse. Good thing I didn't have to shave because it would have made me look even worse. Fortunately, I didn't have to shave then because no hair grew on my face yet. One of the medics asked me what I was there for and where I came from. I tried to explain to him why I was there but my tongue hit against my tooth and made it too painful to talk. The medic called over a few more GI medics. They started to ask me the same thing about where I had come from. I tried so hard to explain to them that I was from the Fifth Division and was there to have the doctor look at my tooth.

They were amazed and kept analyzing me. They were bewildered and asked me so many questions, wanting to know how I endured the life of an infantryman. I told them that I had worn the same clothes for over two months without a bath of any kind. I told the medic that this is what I looked liked for months. They also asked how I slept with all of the shelling and gunfire. They wanted to know if I slept in a house. I explained to them that I slept in foxholes with the mud, rain and freezing cold. I tried so hard to explain to them what it was like up front, but my tooth hurt so badly. It was difficult for the medics to understand me. They looked at me as if I came from the planet Mars. They shook their heads and said, "Oh my

God." with looks of amazement.

One of the medics asked me if I would like something to eat. I asked for some soup. I hadn't eaten since the night before. He came back with a can of soup and some fresh bread. When the medic opened the can of soup with a key, it automatically started to heat up by itself. I asked how it worked and they said the British made it. I wished we had that type of soup up front. After eating the soup, ever so carefully, because of the pain in my tooth, the medic gave me some new clothes and told me to go into the bath house. Someone took me there. I undressed and had a good time taking a shower. It felt so good, warm water and soap! It sure was better than washing out of my helmet.

I put on the new clothes and went to the dentist, who was waiting for me. He had seen me come in earlier all covered in mud from his office. He looked me over and asked me the same questions that the GIs asked me in the hallway. I am sure the GIs told him what I said to them about combat. He looked into my mouth. I pointed out the bad tooth and he told me that it was infected. He gave me some pills to take, but said it was too swollen to pull the tooth out that day and he would have another look at it in the morning. It was badly infected.

The men gave me a canvas cot to sleep on. When I fell asleep, it was like heaven, so peaceful. The medic gave me a few aspirin before going to sleep. I slept so well. There were no enemy guns to worry about. I felt like I was back home in the States. The next morning, I got up and washed and cleaned myself. Then, I had a canteen cup of coffee.

After drinking down the coffee, I went in to see the dentist. I sat in the chair and the dentist gave me a few injections in my gums. After my mouth was numb, he pulled the infected tooth. Then he put a sterile pad on the part which had once been a tooth. He was going to make me a partial and said, "Lots of luck Lauria. I hope you make it through this war."

All of the boys who looked after me while I was there also wished me all the luck in the world. I thanked them and said I could use it. I got back on the truck for the ride back to the front lines. They waved to me as we pulled away. The ride back was quiet and calm. It wasn't going to be peaceful for long. It was only a short time before I heard the sound of artillery and machine gun fire and I started to get afraid again. The day I spent in the rear was like a dream, and it had come to an end.

At least I got a good night sleep and some clean clothes to wear. It only took a couple of days until the new clothes looked as bad as the ones that I left back at the aid station. The dentist made me an impression of my mouth to fit a partial plate. The plate arrived about a month later and I learned to wear them.

I arrived at my company command post and some of the troops greeted me. The outfit advanced a few miles while I was gone. They did a good job without me ha, ha. I was happy to be back with my outfit for one reason. Many of the men that got wounded would never get back to their outfit. Sometimes the army screwed up and sent them somewhere else. After being in my outfit for two years, I had grown attached. This was my home away from home. [lxxii]

1. Did Lauria go to see a dentist immediately after he hurt his tooth?   YES   NO

2. Did they have automatic heated soup up on the front lines?   YES   NO

3. Did Lauria's top Sergeant give him the okay to go see a dentist?   YES   NO

4. Was the closest dentist about 2 miles from the front lines?   YES   NO

5. Was Lauria old enough to need to shave?   YES   NO

6. Did he get the partial place about a month later?   YES   NO

7. Was he happy to get a shower and new clothes?   YES   NO

8. Were the medics used to seeing men from the front lines?   YES   NO

9. Were wounded men always reunited with their original units?   YES   NO

10. What Division was Lauria a part of?

11. How long had he worn the clothes he was in when he got to the dentist?

12. On the front lines, what did Lauria use to hold water to wash himself?

Comprehension of Short Stories

Excerpt from *My Brother the River* by Charles Lytton

Shock of a Lifetime

One time, Daddy and me had a part-time job. After I outgrew well-drilling, we went to work cleaning and maintaining telephone booths. Every Saturday and Sunday this job took us all over the county. Again, the main focus was to keep my mind occupied and my body busy. Daddy didn't care one bit what I was doing, as long as I was busy. At the time, there were telephone booths all over this county. We would just pull up in the parking lot in front of the telephone booth, and I'd wash each window, check the light bulbs and make some repairs.

This one day we show up at the Marina Bridge, on the shore of Claytor Lake. There is a big box and a bunch of aluminum pieces in a pile. I get to looking around and see there is also a little square concrete pad with an electrical wire sticking out of it. I learn that we are going to make a telephone booth. It isn't hard. I empty out the box and start putting the pieces together like a big aluminum puzzle. Within two hours I am standing up on the top of the newly assembled telephone booth, mounting the telephone sign.

Now, Daddy decides not to take a real active part. Up to this point he has been inside drinking coffee, looking at the boats and other things. He wants to see if the electricity has been turned on. He goes into the building and flips the breaker. Please keep in mind that I am standing on top of the booth mounting the light fixture when Pap turns on the power. I am shocked so bad that I fall off.

My whole body is hurting and just trembling and I'm a-screaming. Everyone from the store, marina and parking lot comes running to my aid. Some might have swum from across the lake. About this time, Daddy comes out of the basement and starts hollering at me, "The very first minute I turn my back, you quit on me. You know I can't take my eyes off of you. I will never get this job done if you keep goofing off and setting there on the ground. We got work to do."

My small crowd of concerned people just slowly walks away and says not one word. In a minute or two, I stop twitching and jerking. The screams have stopped, and I am back to kind of mumbling in an unknown language. So I just climb back up on top of the telephone booth; but only after I go into the basement and put the electrical fuses in my pocket. Daddy goes back to drinking coffee and looking around. Some things never change. [lxxiii]

1. What did the author and his Daddy have a job fixing and building?

2. Did his Daddy help him build the telephone booth?

3. What was the name of the lake where he built the telephone booth?

4. What did his Daddy do while he worked?

5. What happened to the author when his Daddy switched the breaker?

6. Was his Daddy sympathetic?

7. Do you think his Daddy knew what had happened?

8. What did the author do to make sure he didn't get shocked again?

Comprehension of Short Stories

Excerpt from *The View from the White Rock* by Charles Lytton
Friends Just be Watchful

All I am saying is just keep your eyes on your friends. You just never know what is going through their evil minds. No sir, you just never know. It is the summer of 1968. Chuck, Jimmy and me are picking up hay on the Obenchain Farm, just outside of Blacksburg. It is just a little hotter than three kinds of hell, and the water in the gallon jug is warm and in limited supply. It is so hot that I have left my best pipe on the dashboard of Chuck's old Ford truck.

After a while, all of the wagons and trucks are loaded, and it is time to start for the barn. I climb in the cab of the truck with Chuck and Jimmy. They are both real quiet, a little too quiet. It is just too hot to talk, so I pick up my old pipe, hold a match over the bowl and draw down deep. Damn this tobacco is strong and right down nasty. It won't stay lit either. I cough a few times, then put a match over the bowl a second time. I suck on the stem real hard. I say, "Damn! Leaving this pipe out in the hot sun has made the tobacco go bad."

About this time both Chuck and Jimmy start to laugh. Not just a chuckle either; it is a deep-down gut-wrenching laugh that just would not stop. I sit there looking at them. I have no clue what the joke is, so I go back to trying to get my pipe to light. The laughter just gets worse. After a few minutes, everything settles down and they tell me they have knocked the tobacco out of my pipe and filled it with dried-up Japanese beetles from the truck's dash.

Yep, keep your eyes on your friends. You just never know what is going through their evil minds. The worst part of this is every summer since smoking them Japanese beetles, I have had a strong urge to eat the leaves off of grape vines.[lxxiv]

1. What town is the farm near?

Springfield   Baldwin   Christiansburg   Blacksburg

2. What year does the story take place?

1998   1968   1966   1958

3. What were the boys doing on the farm?

picking grapes   fixing a tractor   picking apples   picking up hay

4. What was the weather like?

rainy   windy   humid   hot

5. What are the names of the author's friends? (circle two)

Chip   John   Chuck   Jimmy

6. Where did he leave his pipe while they worked?

barn   grass   back of truck   truck's dashboard

7. What did Chuck and Jimmy put in his pipe?

hay   tobacco   Japanese Beetles   crickets

8. From the story, what can we infer that Japanese Beetles eat?

hay   grape leaves   tobacco   wine

Comprehension of Short Stories

Excerpt from *The View from the White Rock* by Charles Lytton

An Interesting Drink

I have to tell you about one of the funniest mixed drinks I ever experienced. Yes, experience is truly what it was. Who were the participants? Chuck Shorter and Waitsie Winters for two, me for three. There were others, but their names have slipped into the last 45 years. I do not recall how it arrived or from where it came, but all of a sudden we were the owners of a brand new, never-been opened, half gallon of store bought vodka. The good stuff; it still had the label on the bottle and everything. Its origin is still a mystery. It is not relevant to the story anyway.

What I do remember is that we took the bottle to Chuck's log cabin on the farm. Waitsie was older and knew how to properly mix vodka into a good mixed drink . You know, kind of like town boys do. After this day I would forever question his knowledge and skills related to alcohol. Chuck rummaged through the cabin and found up a package of "Leftie Lemon". In my day, everyone drank Kool Aid. Lefty Lemon was a knock-off version of Kool Aid.

Chuck finds the Lefty Lemon and a gallon jar. He goes to the creek and gets about a half gallon of water. Then he pours the Lefty Lemon into the jar. Waitsie then stirs in about a pound or more of sugar. Once the Lefty Lemon and sugar are dissolved, Waitsie slowly stirs in the vodka. When the gallon jar is about full, a small sip of this wonderful concoction is poured for us to taste.

The mixture is so sweet it is sickening. You are supposed to get sick the day after you drink the stuff, not when you taste it. Everyone starts to look at Chuck and Waitsie with a very discriminating eye. They start to review the recipe and the mixture. It is discovered the "Leftie Lemon" is the presweetened kind. The mixture has been double sweetened. There is nothing to do but sour it back up. Chuck goes to the cabinet and brings out a bottle of apple cider vinegar. They start adding in a little vinegar, and slowly but surely the mixture becomes sour. Everyone gets a glass full.

Now to be quite honest here, I was grateful for the vodka; well I think I was. Everyone had a great laugh at the look of Chuck's face when the mistake was discovered. But there was still a very funny taste about this mixed drink. My advice to you novice mixers is: do not use creek water or just any old jar from the sideboard. Rinse the jar out a few times![lxxv]

1. Is "Leftie Lemon" a cheaper version of "Kool Aid"?   YES   NO

2. Was Waitsie the youngest one in the group?   YES   NO

3. Was the vodka a gallon bottle?   YES   NO

4. Was the "Leftie Lemon" presweetened?   YES   NO

5. Did they use lemon juice to sour it back up?   YES   NO

6. Did they wash the jug out before they filled it with water?   YES   NO

7. Did they use creek water to make the mixed drink?   YES   NO

8. Was it typical for the boys to have store bought liquor   YES   NO

9. Did the boys live in town?   YES   NO

10. Did they add over a pound of sugar to the mixed drink?   YES   NO

Processing: Level I: Have the patient repeat the word list back in order.
Level II: Have the patient repeat the words back in order but make them plural
Level III: Have the patient repeat the words in reverse order
Level IV: Repeat the words back in alphabetical order

1. Dog   Cat   Guinea Pig

2. Shoe   Hat   Paper towel

3. Phone   Computer   Pencil

4. Watch   Envelope   Yarn

5. Airplane   Bus   Banana

6. Beagle   Zipper   Wallet

7. Eraser   Card   Pretzel

8. Stamp   Bowl   Truck

9. Paper   Backpack   Lunchbox

10. Ring   Nail   Fingernail

11. Tooth   Umbrella   Towel

12. Window   Book   Camera

13. Stair   Tree   Checkbook

14. Bell   Truck   Card

15. Sled   Shovel   Ape

16. Toe   Elbow   Hand

17. Pen   Marker   Apple

18. Flower   Shrub   Dirt

19. Leaf   Photo   Spoon

20. Diamond   Pear   Sock

Processing: Level I: Read the numbers aloud and have the patient repeat the numbers
Level II: Repeat the numbers and add the last two digits together (2363 = 239)
Level II: Add the first two and the last two numbers together (2363 = 59)

1. 2259

2. 1388

3. 3721

4. 5572

5. 4558

6. 7319

7. 7172

8. 2363

9. 9025

10. 1884

11. 1973

12. 1451

13. 3568

14. 6472

15. 6998

16. 3441

17. 3758

18. 7732

19. 2553

20. 8182

Processing: Level I: Repeat the zip code
Level II: Repeat the zip code in reverse order
Level III: Repeat the zip code and add the last two numbers (24061 = 2407)

1. 71149

2. 19731

3. 23462

4. 28277

5. 19350

6. 71355

7. 90212

8. 91042

9. 94114

10. 10179

11. 60613

12. 59820

13. 80942

14. 54712

15. 18361

16. 28105

17. 53622

18. 17399

19. 90225

20. 11731

Processing: Level I: Repeat the phone number
Level II: Repeat it back but add 1 to the last digit 541 8224= 541 8225
Level II: Repeat the phone number backwards 541 8224 = 4228 145

1. 862 5391

2. 542 6603

3. 328 0106

4. 612 5834

5. 708 5304

6. 246 3555

7. 222 4357

8. 544 0131

9. 268 3442

10. 542 9159

11. 491 8199

12. 234 6064

13. 845 2742

14. 296 9898

15. 333 4130

16. 849 7238

17. 572 9782

18. 589 4885

19. 843 4100

20. 254 8022

Calculation

1. Soup was on sale for 10 for $10. I bought twenty cans how much did they all cost?

2. Frozen meals cost $2.50 a piece. I have a coupon for $2.00 off if I buy 6. How much will 6 frozen meals cost if I use my coupon?

3. I had a gift card to Target for $50. The items I bought cost a total of $68. How much money in addition to the gift card will I need?

4. My cell phone plan costs $40 a month. How much does it cost a year?

5. Tammy went on a diet and after 6 months lost 35 lbs. She was very happy with her new weight of 150 lbs. What did she weigh before she started her diet?

6. I rented a car for 4 days for $30 a day. How much was the total?

7. He made $50,000 a year. Taxes took 20%. How much did he get to keep?

8. Trash bags cost $3 a box. They were on sale for buy 2 get 3 free. How much did 5 boxes cost?

9. The champion Golden Retriever had a litter of 6 puppies. 2 boys and 4 girls. Girls cost $1000 each and the boys cost $750 each. How much did the litter cost?

10. The pharmacy closed at 6 pm. It was 8:30 pm. How long had the pharmacy been closed?

11. He had $10,000 in credit card debt at a 15% yearly APR. How much would he have to pay in interest a year?

12. A Mom and Dad took their two children to the movies. Adult tickets were $8.50 a piece and a ticket for a child was $6 a piece. How much did all 4 tickets cost?

13. The same family purchased snacks at the movies. They bought one large popcorn for $8, 1 box of M&Ms for $4, and 4 medium sodas for $2.50 each. How much did their snack order cost?

14. How much did their outing to the movies cost all together?

15. Kate spent $150 a week on groceries for her family. How much was their monthly grocery bill?

16. Doctors recommend you drink half your body weight in water in ounces. Tom weighed 200 lbs. How many ounces of water should he drink a day?

17. A couple bought a fixer-upper house for $300,000. They spent $100,000 on renovations. When they finished, they sold the home for $550,000. How much did they make in profit?

18. Before the recession, Paul bought a home for $800,000 near Washington, DC. A year after the housing bubble burst, the value of his home dropped to $575,000. How much did the value of the home depreciate?

19. Kate was used to going to the dermatologist 4 times a year. She spent $120 per visit including medication to control her acne. She was considering switching to a popular skin regiment to prevent acne that cost $40 a month instead of regularly seeing the dermatologist. How much does each option cost a year and which one is cheaper?

20. Newlyweds booked a hotel in Waikiki, Hawaii for 10 nights for $250 a night. Their flights to Honolulu cost $750 a piece and the car rental was $50 a day. How much would their honeymoon cost?

21. He had $3,500 to spend to renovate his basement. Carpet cost $2,000, paint and supplies cost $300 and a new bathroom vanity cost $500. How much did he spend and was he under budget?

22. The grocery store has a special this week that doubles the value of coupons. I had coupons for $1.50 off 5 cans of soup, $1.00 off 6 frozen meals, 50 cents off paper towels and $2.00 off vitamins. How much was my total savings in coupons?

23. She had her car washed every other month and spent $20 on the deluxe package. How much did she spend a year on car washes?

24. Dog food cost $35 for a 40lb bag. The pet supply store had a sale for 20% off all dog food bags over 20lbs. What did the bag of dog food cost after the discount?

25. The babysitter charges $15 an hour. The parents went out for their anniversary and were gone for 5 hours. How much did they need to pay the babysitter?

26. Sally went to the hair dresser once a month. It cost $50 to get her hair cut and colored. The salon had a promotion after 10 appointments you get one free. How much did she spend a year at the salon?

27. Tom lived in a rural area and trash removal cost him $40 every three months. How much did he spend in a year?

28. Dinner at a nice restaurant for the family cost $150. If a 20% tip was added, how much was the final bill?

29. A birthday party at a skating rink cost $10 per child plus $25 for the party room and $30 for a cake. If 10 children attended, how much would the party cost?

30. County property taxes had cost Bob $300 a year. This year there is a 5% tax increase. How much are his new taxes?

31. Mary and Jim joined a gym for $60 a month for a couple. How much did it cost them for a year?

32. There was a sale on vitamins for buy one, get one half off. If you bought two bottles of calcium that normally were $15 a piece, how much did you spend with the sale?

33. Hank's annual home insurance premium was $600 if he paid it all at once. If he switched to monthly payments, it would cost him $1 more each month. What would his monthly payment be?

34. Four college students decided to rent a house. The monthly rental was $1200. How much would it cost each student each month?

35. Tommy received $50 for his birthday from his grandparents. He decided to buy some toy cars which cost $8 each. How many cars could he buy and how much money did he have left over?

36. Mary weighed 180 pounds. She went on a diet and started exercising and lost 1/3 of her body weight. How much weight did she lose?

37. Dave drives 15 miles each way to and from work. How many total miles does he drive to and from work Monday-Friday?

38. The average high temperature in January is 35 degrees. Today the temperature was 20% lower than average. What was the temperature today?

39. Rose bushes usually cost $20. The garden center had a sale – buy one, get one free. If I bought a dozen rose bushes on sale, how much did I pay?

40. A class of children decided to color Easter eggs. They had five dozen eggs and colored 10% green, 20% yellow, 30% purple and 40% blue. How many eggs were there of each color?

41. Jenny was paid $10 a day to feed a neighbor's cat while they were on vacation for a week. How much did she earn?

42. Susan and Bob usually used 25,000 air miles each to fly to visit their daughter in Texas, but to make the trip during the Christmas holiday it would cost them double the usual miles. How many air miles did they need for both of them to make the fly to Texas at Christmas time?

43. The grocery store lets me earn money off the price of gasoline. If I earned 40 cents off per gallon and I bought 15 gallons of gas, how much did I save?

44. After Christmas, I went to the mall to spend some gift cards and Christmas cash during the post holiday sales. At one store I bought a sweater for $22, a pair of slacks for $37 and a blouse for $18. I used a $50 gift card to pay part of the bill. How much cash did I need to spend?

45. One morning Linda decided to run several errands. She drove 4 miles to the post office to buy some stamps. She then drove 2 miles to the bank to deposit a check. Next she drove ½ mile to the library to return a book. Then she drove 1 ½ miles to the pharmacy to pick up a prescription. Finally she drove 3 miles to the grocery store to pick up a few items. She then drove 6 miles home. How many miles did she drive that morning?

46. Jennifer's class sold popcorn as a fundraiser. Each box cost them $1 and they sold them for $2. Jennifer sold 25 boxes, Adam sold 35 boxes, Karen sold 50 boxes and the rest of the class sold a total of 270 boxes. How much profit did the class make?

47. Tony used wood stoves to help heat his house. Most years he used 8 cords of wood that cost him $100 per cord. The past winter was much colder than normal and he used 10 cords of wood which cost him $150 per cord. How much more did he spend on firewood last year than in a normal year?

48. Frank had a comic book collection that he decided to sell. He sold 50 comic books for $10 each, 5 for $20 each, 10 for $30 each and 10 for $50 each. What was the total amount that he made from the sale?

49. Steve decided to hike part of the Appalachian Trail during his summer vacation. He planned to take 20 days to hike a 180 mile section of the trail. How many miles did he need to hike each day to reach his goal?

50. Margaret loved going to her library's used book sale. On opening day, she bought 3 premium books for $3 each, 1 premium book for $10, 15 regular hardback books for $1 each and 6 paperback books for $.50 each. On the final day she bought two bags of books for $6.50 a bag. How much did she spend?

51. June had been looking at a winter coat at the mall that originally cost $200. She waited to purchase it until the coat was on sale for 75% off. How much did she pay for the coat?

52. Ruth had three daughters, who each had three daughters, who each had three daughters. How many great-granddaughters did Ruth have?

Calculation Answer Key

1. $20
2. $13
3. $18
4. $480
5. 185 lbs
6. $120
7. $40,000
8. $6
9. $5,500
10. Two and a half hours
11. $1500
12. $29
13. $22
14. $51
15. $600
16. 100 oz
17. $150,000
18. $225,000
19. They both cost $480 a year
20. $4500
21. $2800, yes
22. $10
23. $120
24. $28
25. $75
26. $550
27. $160
28. $180
29. $155
30. $315
31. $720
32. $22.50
33. $51
34. $300
35. 6 cars $2 left over
36. 60lbs
37. 150 miles
38. 28 degrees
39. $120
40. 6 green 12 yellow 18 purple 24 blue
41. $70

42. 100,000 air miles
43. $6
44. $27
45. 17 miles
46. $380
47. $700
48. $1400
49. 9 miles a day
50. $50
51. $50
52. 27 great-granddaughters

i   Source: European Southern Observatory, CC-BY, via: http://www.eso.org/public/images/eso0848a/

ii   Source: Booyabazooka, CC-BY, via: http://commons.wikimedia.org/wiki/File:Cat_silhouette.svg

iii Source: Amada44, CC-BY, via: http://commons.wikimedia.org/wiki/File:Dog_Silhouette_01.svg

iv Source Andreas06, CC-BY, via:: http://commons.wikimedia.org/wiki/File:Sinnbild_Kraftomnibus.svg

v   Source: Andreas06, CC-BY, via: http://commons.wikimedia.org/wiki/File:Zusatzzeichen_1006-37.svg

vi Source: Andreas06, CC-BY, via: http://commons.wikimedia.org/wiki/File:Sinnbild_Tiere.svg

vii Source: Andreas06, CC-BY, via: http://commons.wikimedia.org/wiki/File:Sinnbild_PKW.svg

viii Source: Andreas06, CC-BY, via:http://commons.wikimedia.org/wiki/File:Sinnbild_Autobahnkiosk.svg

ix Source: Andreas06, CC-BY, via:http://commons.wikimedia.org/wiki/File:Zusatzzeichen_1010-11.svg

x   Source: MarianSigler, CC-BY, via: http://commons.wikimedia.org/wiki/File:Sinnbild_Radfahrer.svg

xi Source: Andreas06, CC-BY, via: http://commons.wikimedia.org/wiki/File:Sinnbild_Traktor.svg

xii Source: Andreas06, CC-BY, via: http://commons.wikimedia.org/wiki/File:Zusatzzeichen_1046-12.svg

xiii Source: Andreas06, CC-BY, via: http://commons.wikimedia.org/wiki/File:Sinnbild_Reiter.svg

xiv Source: Mediatus, CC-BY, via: http://commons.wikimedia.org/wiki/File:Sinnbild_Sch%C3%BClerlotsen.png

xv Source: Qualle, CC-BY, via: http://commons.wikimedia.org/wiki/File:Sinnbild_Autobahnhotel.svg

xvi Source:Cmprince. CC-BY via: http://commons.wikimedia.org/wiki/File:Aiga_watertransportation.gif

xvii Source:Cmprince. CC-BY via:http://commons.wikimedia.org/wiki/File:Aiga_departingflights.gif

xviii Source:Cmprince. CC-BY via: http://commons.wikimedia.org/wiki/File:Aiga_fireextinguisher.gif

xix Source:Cmprince. CC-BY via:http://commons.wikimedia.org/wiki/File:Aiga_nursery.gif

xx Source: Alison Wheeler, CC-BY via: http://commons.wikimedia.org/wiki/File:BSicon_HELI.svg

xxi Source: Spolyak68, CC-BY via: http://commons.wikimedia.org/wiki/File:565_Care_Staff_Area.jpg

xxii Source:DieBouche, CC-BY, via: http://commons.wikimedia.org/wiki/File:Symbol_great.svg

xxiii Source:Allstarecho, CC-BY, via: http://commons.wikimedia.org/wiki/File:Cigarette.png

xxiv Source: Nevit Dilmen, CC-BY, via: http://commons.wikimedia.org/wiki/File:2008-07-25_Geese_over_01.svg

xxv Source: George Jansoone, CC-BY, via:
    http://commons.wikimedia.org/wiki/File:Museum_of_Anatolian_Civilizations_100.svg

xxvi Source: Nevit Dilmen, CC-BY, via: http://commons.wikimedia.org/wiki/File:Catty.svg

xxvii Source: Nevit Dilmen, CC-BY, via:http://commons.wikimedia.org/wiki/File:Hirundorusticaflightcropped.svg

xxviii Source: Amada 44, CC-BY, via:http://commons.wikimedia.org/wiki/File:Shark_silhouette.svg

xxix Source: Angelus, CC-BY, via: http://commons.wikimedia.org/wiki/File:Dragon_silhouette.svg

xxx Source: Jcfidy, CC-BY, via: http://commons.wikimedia.org/wiki/File:Chicken_Silhouette.png

xxxi Source: Nekar Jon C, CC-BY, via: http://commons.wikimedia.org/wiki/File:Brachiosaurus_silhouette.svg

xxxii Source: Andreas Plank, CC-BY, via: http://commons.wikimedia.org/wiki/File:Meadow_site_silhouette.svg

xxxiii Source: Andreas Plank, CC-BY, via: http://commons.wikimedia.org/wiki/File:Mixed_forest_silhouette.svg

xxxiv Source: Andreas Plank, CC-BY, via: http://commons.wikimedia.org/wiki/File:Field_site_silhouette.svg

xxxv Source: Andreas Plank, CC-BY, via: http://commons.wikimedia.org/wiki/File:Park_side_silhouette.svg

xxxvi Source: Andreas Plank, CC-BY, via: http://commons.wikimedia.org/wiki/File:High_mountain_region_silhouette.svg

xxxvii Source: Andreas Plank, CC-BY, via: http://commons.wikimedia.org/wiki/File:River_silhouette.svg

xxxviii Source: Andreas Plank, CC-BY, via: http://commons.wikimedia.org/wiki/File:City_silhouette.svg

xxxix Source: Andreas Plank, CC-BY, via: http://commons.wikimedia.org/wiki/File:Lake_silhouette.svg

xl Source: openclipart.org, CC-BY, via: http://commons.wikimedia.org/wiki/File:Karate_silhouette.svg

xli Source: Slomoc, CC-BY, via: http://commons.wikimedia.org/wiki/File:Stevel_silhouette.svg

xlii Source: Nevit Dilmen, CC-BY, via: http://commons.wikimedia.org/wiki/File:Silhouette_1330283.svg

xliii Source: Nevit Dilmen, CC-BY, via: http://commons.wikimedia.org/wiki/File:Silhouette_1330244.svg

xliv Source: Calvito Mallory, CC-BY, via:http://commons.wikimedia.org/wiki/File:CalvitoMallory.svg

xlv Source: Nevit Dilmen, CC-BY, via: http://commons.wikimedia.org/wiki/File:Silhouette_1330347a.svg

xlvi Source: Nevit Dilmen, CC-BY, via: http://commons.wikimedia.org/wiki/File:Gymnastics-bw.svg

xlvii Source: Nevit Dilmen, CC-BY, via: http://commons.wikimedia.org/wiki/File:Silhouette_1330285.svg

xlviii Source: Nevit Dilmen, CC-BY, via: http://commons.wikimedia.org/wiki/File:Skoczek.svg

xlix Source: Carstor, CC-BY, via: http://commons.wikimedia.org/wiki/File:Downhill_sketch.svg

l   Source: Kalka, CC-BY, via:http://commons.wikimedia.org/wiki/File:Break_dance.svg

li   Source: Nevit Dilmen, CC-BY, via: http://commons.wikimedia.org/wiki/File:Kalymnos_2005_022.svg

lii Source: Phil Bronnery CC-BY, via: http://commons.wikimedia.org/wiki/File:2Silhouette_Female.jpg

liii Source: Alexander Kiko, CC-BY, via: http://commons.wikimedia.org/wiki/File:Band_Silhouette_04.jpg

liv Source: Alexander Kiko, CC-BY, via: http://commons.wikimedia.org/wiki/File:Band_Silhouette_01.svg

lv Source: Alexander Kiko, CC-BY, via: http://commons.wikimedia.org/wiki/File:Band_Silhouette_05.svg

lvi Source: Inkwina, CC-BY, via: http://commons.wikimedia.org/wiki/File:Car_with_Driver-Silhouette.svg

lvii Source: Andreas Plank, CC-BY, via: http://commons.wikimedia.org/wiki/File:Mixed_forest_silhouette_scaled-tohight,_quadratic.svg

lviii Source: Rama, CC-BY, via:
http://commons.wikimedia.org/wiki/File:De_Havilland_DH_60.GIII_Moth_Major_img_0504-silhouette.svg Rama

lix Source: Onef9day, CC-BY, via:http://commons.wikimedia.org/wiki/File:Silhouette_yoga.png

lx Source: Onef9day, CC-BY, via: http://commons.wikimedia.org/wiki/File:Coat_Silhouette.svg

lxi Source: Spedona, CC-BY, via:http://commons.wikimedia.org/wiki/File:H
%C3%A9raldique_meuble_Feuille_de_vigne.svg

lxii Source: Twisp, CC-BY, via: http://commons.wikimedia.org/wiki/File:Wineglass.svg Twisp

lxiii Source: Lionel Allorge, CC-BY, via:http://commons.wikimedia.org/wiki/File:Flower01.svg

lxiv Source: Ian Burt CC-BY, via: http://commons.wikimedia.org/wiki/File:Salix_fragilis_Silhouette_(oddsock).png Ian
Burt

lxv Source: Zaidaudi, CC-BY, via:http://commons.wikimedia.org/wiki/File:Floor_Plan.pdf

lxvi Source: RTCNCA, CC-BY, via: http://commons.wikimedia.org/wiki/File:Whitehouse_street_map.svg

lxvii Source: Bjs, CC-BY, via: http://commons.wikimedia.org/wiki/File:Grundriss_Couvenmuseum_Erdgeschoss.png

lxviii Source: CC-BY, via: http://en.wikipedia.org/wiki/Morphine

lxix http://en.wikipedia.org/wiki/Chocolate_chip_cookie

lxx Lauria, Louis, J. *Running Wire at the Front Lines,* Jefferson, NC: McFarland, 2011.

lxxi Lauria, Louis, J. *Running Wire at the Front Lines,* Jefferson, NC: McFarland, 2011.

lxxii Lauria, Louis, J. *Running Wire at the Front Lines,* Jefferson, NC: McFarland, 2011.

lxxiii Lytton, Charles, *My Brother the River,* Blacksburg, VA. Pennyworth LLC. 2013.

lxxiv Lytton, Charles, *The View From the White Rock,* Charleston SC. Pennyworth LLC. 2012.

lxxv Lytton, Charles, *The View From the White Rock,* Charleston SC. Pennyworth LLC. 2012.

Printed in Great Britain
by Amazon

19068729R00093